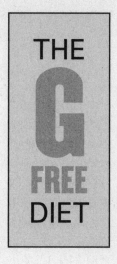

THE
G
FREE
DIET

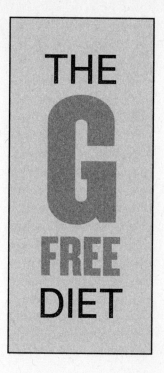

THE G FREE DIET

A GLUTEN-FREE SURVIVAL GUIDE

ELISABETH HASSELBECK

with a Foreword by Peter Green, MD

CENTER
STREET

NEW YORK BOSTON NASHVILLE

This book is not intended as a substitute for the medical advice of physicians. The reader should regularly consult a physician in all matters relating to his or her health, and particularly with respect to any symptoms that may require diagnosis or medical attention.

Center Street
Hachette Book Group
237 Park Avenue
New York, NY 10017

www.centerstreet.com

Center Street is a division of Hachette Book Group, Inc.
The Center Street name and logo are trademarks of Hachette Book Group, Inc.

Printed in the United States of America

Originally published in hardcover by Center Street.

First Trade Edition: January 2011
10 9 8 7 6 5 4 3 2 1

The Library of Congress has cataloged the hardcover edition as follows:
Hasselbeck, Elisabeth.
  The G-free diet : a gluten-free survival guide / Elisabeth Hasselbeck. — 1st ed.
    p. cm.
  ISBN 978-1-59995-188-1
  1. Gluten-free diet—Popular works.   2. Celiac disease—Popular works.   I. Title.
  RM237.86.H37 2009
  613.2'5—dc22
                                                                    2008053768

ISBN 978-1-59995-189-8 (pbk.)

To Mama—
You are missed.
You are loved.
You are always with us.

CONTENTS

ACKNOWLEDGMENTS

It has been a long road to recovery and renewed sense of health. More than ten years of research, blood work, testing, uncertainty, pain, and trial by fire will be put to good use, as my hope is that this book will be a resource for those who are already, and those who are on their way to being, G-free. This book was made possible by a desire to channel all of those years together, the willingness to look forward, and a remarkable team of individuals around me. Thank you for reading the book, trusting that the G-free diet is right for you, and joining me as I acknowledge those who helped make this book happen.

Truly, a most special thanks to Dr. Peter Green, for taking the time to investigate what was really happening with my digestive system, for being kind enough to lend your wisdom to *The G-Free Diet*, both in the body of the book and in the Foreword. The community and support at the Celiac Disease Center is tremendously appreciated. Your good work is a gift to us all. Many thanks for helping so many regain health, and for putting the faith we place in you to great work.

A most meaningful thanks to my newfound friend Laura Moser—a most talented writer, soon-to-be mom, and novelist! Thank you for reading my countless midnight e-mails, for keeping me on schedule, and for your equally matched diligence and zeal while working with me. I wish you the most joyous transition into motherhood, and look forward to reading your future masterpiece!

I cannot thank Center Street Publishing and the rest of the Hachette Book Group enough for believing in me. A highlighted thanks to my most thorough and thoughtful editor, Michelle Rapkin, for understanding the passion that I have for this subject matter. My thanks to the entire team for supporting me throughout the process, for the chance to put my decade-plus of research and writing to good use, and for opening your arms to *The G-Free Diet*.

A great amount of appreciation goes to Dr. Kenneth Bock, Ashley Koff, and Dr. Andrew Weil for their expert advice, astuteness, information, and time spent with me throughout the course of writing this book. I value our conversations, as they were filled with the dedication you have to those who seek your help. Your work with others to make lives more whole, complete, and healthy is without a doubt a vocation that we can all be thankful for. I admire each of you for taking the road less traveled. Ashley, your meal suggestions are fantastic and delicious.

He hears me say it every time a workout session is over—but not enough as far as I am concerned: Pat Manocchia, founder of the Center for Preventative Medicine and La Palestra in NYC, I thank you for revamping my workouts, and your constant commitment to absolute integration of body, nutrition, and mind. Thank you for making my workouts hard, and my life much easier.

To the wonderfully honest, open, and warm Kathy Burger, Rose and Peter Miller, and Patrick Cole, for sharing with me your G-free journey, I thank you. I appreciate every phone call and e-mail that you made to make this book real for so many others. Those who can visualize your paths will find comfort that, for whatever reason, being G-free can work for them, too. I cannot thank you enough.

Babette Perry, my broadcasting agent of nearly a decade, thank you for being a most wonderful confidant, friend, and sounding board. Thank you for always honoring my "gut" instinct, for my calls at all hours, and for being such a wonderful role model as a working mom and wife. Your work is outstanding.

A huge thanks to my literary agent, Andrea Barzvi, for being the first to get the G-free bug, for understanding my unbridled enthusiasm, for your patience, and for your unending support throughout this process. We got there! Your guidance has been spot-on.

Applause to my sensational licensing team, Tim Rothwell, Zoe Anne Murphy, Michael Gotssegan, and Lisa Mitchell. You have been sharply instrumental in allowing my designs and products to come to life. An all-star team indeed! Thanks to my commercial agents, Karen Sellars and Jason Pinyan, for continued work on my behalf, and for great loyalty over the years.

A warm thanks to ABC Television, Bill Geddie, and Barbara Walters, for respecting my voice and offering me the chance of a lifetime. To Barbara Walters, Whoopi Goldberg, Joy Behar, Sherri Shepherd, Karl Nilsson, Jordana Kalmanowitz, Karen Dupiche, Lavette Slater, Rebecca Borman, Rosa Amoedo, and our entire production staff and crew at *The View*—who carefully watch everything I eat, drink, wear, and use on my face and hair on and off the set to be certain that it is G-free—I thank you all! A great thanks, as well, to my colorist, Keith Bocklett, and his team for checking that every label and product that I come in contact with at the salon is G-free! (And for keeping my roots at bay!) To all of my friends who constantly look out for me when out to eat, or visiting...I love you all.

Many thanks to so many viewers who have come to the show, watched, or written to me about their battle with celiac disease—I hope that this provides comfort, strategy, and some laughs. A note of appreciation, as well, to the many companies that have recognized the importance and need for G-free facilities and food. I thank you from the bottom of my belly!

A most special thank-you to my entire family: Mom, Dad, Kenny, Betsy, Don, Matthew, Sarah, Nathanael: Thank you for being my Gluten Guards. For all that you have done for me through words, deeds, and prayer, I thank you, and I love you all.

For my husband, Tim, countless thanks for your commitment and support over the years. Thank you for wiping the pretzels off your mouth before kissing me. I love you. Always have. Always will.

Grace, my little G-free guardian: Thank you for asking me, "Mommy, is that G-free?" when I am about to eat something, because I know your little heart is concerned about me getting a hurt tummy. Thanks for baking and taste-testing my G-free treats with me, and for being the affectionate, caring, and loving big sister you are. I love you to the moon and back!

Taylor, I love you and will take your kisses full of graham cracker crumbs any day! Thank you for loving me so. You are becoming such a strong little man.

For our little one on the way, I thank you for filling my days and nights with joy and anticipation, and for letting me indulge in even *more* G-free treats! I love you already.

FOREWORD

Many people wonder why I became so interested in celiac disease. In fact, it started many years ago in my medical training in Australia. We were taught that the disease was common, occurred mainly in adults, and people did not have to have diarrhea. I have merely been practicing what I learned during my excellent medical training in Australia. I needed to travel overseas to obtain further research experience with a view of returning to Australia. My research into intestinal absorption took me to Harvard Medical School in Boston and then Columbia University in New York, where I have remained.

Because of my original research interest in small intestinal function and absorption, as well as celiac disease, I diagnosed and looked after patients with celiac disease more often than my colleagues. Probably a pivotal point in my celiac disease career was in 1990 when I diagnosed celiac disease in a woman, Sue Goldstein. She subsequently started the Westchester Celiac Support Group in New York. This has since grown into a large independent support group. Sue started suggesting that patients come into New York City to see me for an opinion as to their diagnosis and management. Initially, both of us received calls from local gastroenterologists that we were stealing their patients! However, the result was that I had a large number of patients with celiac disease. This has allowed me to note variations in presentations, increase my experience with this amazing disease, get other physicians and investigators at Columbia interested in the disease, and publish research on the disease. I was surprised to become an expert in this disease. There are probably no other diseases in the United States with fewer "experts."

I started the Celiac Disease Center at Columbia University, with the help of Sue and several other patients, with three goals in mind:

1. To provide excellent medical care for individuals with celiac disease and gluten sensitivity.
2. To perform research into the disease. To help understand the mechanisms that cause the disease and its associated medical conditions as well as the economic impact of the diagnosis.
3. To provide education to patients as well as physicians and other health care workers about celiac disease.

The Center has grown considerably in several years. Patients have come not only from the metropolitan New York City area, but also from all around the country and overseas as well. As a result, there has been a growth in the number of physicians, both pediatric and adult gastroenterologists, joining us to provide care for an increasing number of people. The clinical experience we have all acquired in looking after people with gluten-related problems is very great. This provides enormous benefit to those that are seen in our Center.

In addition, the other goals of the Center are being continually fulfilled. We have a multitude of research papers that highlight the clinical manifestations of the disease as well as the associated conditions and provide insights into the mechanisms of the disease. We have collaborated with leaders in the field from all over the world. This research has helped educate physicians about the disease. It is through physician education that a greater number of patients will be diagnosed and receive appropriate follow-up care. Follow-up medical care of patients with celiac disease is totally lacking in this country. All our research and educational activities have been funded by the generosity of people with celiac disease, their friends and families.

Since the opening of the Celiac Disease Center at Columbia University, research has shown that celiac disease is very common, affecting about 1 percent of the population, and led us to understand the mechanism of this very interesting and life-altering disease. Research has also led us to understand the mechanism of the associated increased rate of many other autoimmune diseases and various malignancies, all of which add a burden of health problems to those with celiac disease. Importantly, a strict G-free diet reduces the risk of the acquisition of both new autoimmune diseases and malignancies. These are great reasons for those who need it to follow a strict G-free diet, and all the more reason for reading Elisabeth's book.

Many people worldwide have adopted a G-free diet. This diet may be lifesaving to those with celiac disease, while others simply find their lives much more comfortable, having found their neurological or gastrointestinal symptoms improved since adopting a G-free lifestyle. Those with dermatitis herpetiformis find their lives now tolerable. Children with autism may improve on a G-free diet, though more scientific studies need to be performed on this topic.

I first met Elisabeth when she came to see me as a patient. She had self-diagnosed celiac disease. We see this often. Usually patients have exhausted their medical providers searching for an answer as to why they feel so terrible. They either look up their symptoms on the Internet or get advice from friends. They work it out! A G-free diet resolves symptoms and restores their health.

In this setting, it can be pretty clear whether someone does or could have celiac disease. Evidence includes the presence of the necessary genes, and usually some evidence of residual vitamin or mineral deficiency. Frequently we find other family members have the disease, further confirming that the original patient was correct. Elisabeth wanted to know about what vitamins she should be taking and about whether her daughter, Grace, and her parents should be tested. People who self-diagnose and treat will usually have normal blood tests for the celiac antibodies, and a normal biopsy, because they have been on the G-free diet for greater than a year.

Those with gluten sensitivity in the absence of celiac disease have a great difficulty getting satisfaction from the medical community. Without an abnormal biopsy, there is difficulty among many physicians accepting such a diagnosis. I, however, regard the diagnosis as valid, providing that celiac disease is excluded. Many of those who have adopted a G-free diet have not had celiac disease excluded. Their self-diagnosis of IBS or gluten sensitivity may, in fact, represent undiagnosed celiac disease.

To understand celiac disease, we need to understand what happens when we (all of us) eat grains containing gluten, the protein component of the cereal grains wheat, rye, and barley. Compared to meat protein, our digestive enzymes cannot digest or degrade gluten protein into its building blocks, the amino acids. It is these larger molecules that exist in all our intestines that are toxic to those that get celiac disease. These molecules enter the lining of the small intestine, probably during gastrointestinal infections, and react with the immune system, causing inflammation. The inflammation causes intestinal villi to atrophy. Instead of the intestine looking like a shag carpet with many little fingers or villi waving in the breeze, it looks more like a regular flat carpet. As a result of the villous atrophy, absorption is reduced. The inflammation results in the release of antibodies and inflammatory proteins into the circulation, affecting the function of many other organs and causing generalized symptoms such as fatigue.

We understand much about why people have celiac disease, but little about nonceliac gluten sensitivity. Probably there is more insight into why people get celiac disease than there is about the other autoimmune conditions. We have as yet to work out why gluten makes others sick in the absence of celiac disease.

The major issue facing us is the underdiagnosis of celiac disease. Underdiagnosis of celiac disease occurs throughout the world. It is, however, most marked in the United States, where it is estimated that less than 5 percent of those with the disease are currently diagnosed. This compares with many countries where awareness of the disease is great. Examples include Finland, where 70 percent of those with the disease are diagnosed. Awareness is great in Australia, Ireland, Italy, and many countries of South America. Great awareness of this disease and gluten sensitivity among the general populations results in an easier life for those on a G-free diet, ready understanding, and easy availability.

Our research has shown that patients may have a long duration of symptoms prior to diagnosis. This includes both children and adults. The delay is not due to the patients failing to seek health care; it is due to physicians failing to consider the diagnosis. This comes down to a failure of physician education on the subject. Generally physicians are not aware of how common the disease actually is, or the best way to diagnose it. Why is this problem exacerbated in the United States? One likely reason is that the pharmaceutical industry has great sway over the direction of medical care in the United States, being responsible for the majority of both medical research and medical education. Celiac disease has received little attention from the pharmaceutical industry because the therapy is dietary, and as a result, until recently there has been little interest in the disease from among the university-based academic centers. However, this is changing. Not only are there a few university-based celiac centers, but there is interest from the pharmaceutical industry as well.

The G-free diet is necessary for those with celiac disease. It prevents the development of symptoms and reverses them when present. The G-free diet improves the quality of life of those with celiac disease and has been shown to reverse osteoporosis, improve the cardiovascular risk profile, reduce the development of autoimmune disease, and prevent the development of cancer in celiac disease patients. For those with gluten sensitivity, the benefits are comfort! All of these are great reasons to eagerly adopt the G-free lifestyle. Read the book and enjoy the diet!

> Peter Green, MD
> Professor of Clinical Medicine
> Director of the Celiac Disease Center
> Columbia University
> New York
> www.celiacdiseasecenter.org

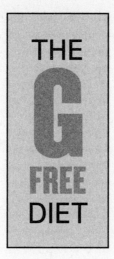

THE
G
FREE
DIET

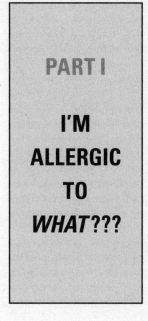

PART I

I'M
ALLERGIC
TO
WHAT???

My G-Free Journey

I learned about gluten the hard way. I wrote this book so you don't have to.

Most people with celiac disease, like me, have a story to tell. My hope is that in reading mine, and the pages that follow, you will be able to begin your journey to a better body and a better self—without all the heartache (and bellyache!) that I endured for far too long.

I grew up in an Italian-American neighborhood in Providence, Rhode Island. There wasn't a single holiday that did not feature "Mama's" (my grandmother's) famous baked penne along with a thirty-inch loaf of fresh Italian bread. After dessert, my whole family would even sit around dunking any remaining bread into our coffee. My cousins and I would fight over who got the "end" of each loaf. I remember watching Mama slice into the loaf, waiting to see if it was my "day" or not.

The smell of more toasted Italian bread and butter would wake me up the next morning.

In my childhood home, it was all bread, all the time—and that was just the way we liked it.

While some things haven't changed in my family—we still have baked penne at every holiday dinner—other things certainly have. Since 2002, for example, my mom has made *two* baked penne: one for everyone else, and one just for me, a gluten-free version that hurts neither my stomach nor Mama's feelings when she looks over and sees a plate devoid of our traditional family fare.

"What do you mean you 'can't have the penne'?" Mama would question me after we sat down at her table. Over and over, I would try to explain to my grandmother, whom I love with my whole heart, and hated to upset at all, that "I am allergic to the pasta."

"Since when?" she would immediately shoot back.

The answer to that was a bit more complicated.

The trouble began in early 1997, during the spring of my sophomore year of college. I went on two big trips that spring. The first, over winter break, was a three-week-long immersion/teaching trip to the village of Red Bank and the city of Dangriga in Belize. The second, a spring training trip, was within the United States, with my Boston College softball team.

I had been feeling a little under the weather since Belize, and shortly after I returned from the softball trip, I was diagnosed with a severe bacterial intestinal infection—residue, the doctor said, from my trip to Central America. I landed in the school infirmary for nearly a week, with an immensely distended belly and a 103- to 104-degree fever. My memories of that week are hazy at best: I can recall little more than opening my eyes to see my mom standing over the bed. And Tim, my college sweetheart and now husband, looking more than concerned.

Once the initial infection had subsided, I was incredibly relieved, thinking I was finally in the clear. As an athlete, I couldn't bear the thought of being "off my game" for more than a day or two. Little did I suspect that my game was going to be significantly "off" for quite some time…

After leaving the infirmary, I was eager to get my body back on track again, but my digestive system was seemingly shot. My efforts to regain some of the muscle mass I had lost during my convalescence went nowhere. And though I felt ravenously hungry *all the time*, the only dining hall option that looked even remotely appetizing to me was soft-serve vanilla frozen yogurt with Rice Krispies mixed in. Food just didn't appeal to me like it had before.

Regardless, I continued to eat, though nothing satisfied my hunger—and everything seemed to throw my stomach into a frenzy. Each meal left me bloated and gassy, with sharp, explosive pains in my abdomen. No matter what I ate, I would soon be doubled over with cramps, awful indigestion, diarrhea—or all of the above simultaneously. I soon became all too familiar with the location of any and all bathrooms. Half an hour later, I would be too lethargic to move.

What on earth was happening to me? I had always been filled with energy before, and now I wanted to crawl back into bed five times a day. I was always in pain, always uncomfortable—especially around mealtimes.

Food, for the first time to this pasta-loving girl, had become the enemy. I was at war with my own body, and it soon became obvious that I was losing each and every battle.

Early on, I (and everyone around me) attributed my difficulties to stress, combined with a lingering infection in my gut. But as time went on and I made my first career move out of school—working as a footwear designer for PUMA—my health only worsened. I was barely able to get through the day without being sideswiped by extreme pain and overwhelming fatigue. I would retreat to the bathroom every ten minutes or so, locking myself in a stall and pressing on my belly in an effort to get control of the spastic bouts in my intestinal region. To keep my colleagues from suspecting that I was under the weather *all the time*, I would strategically walk a different way to the ladies' room each time, to avoid passing the same person twice in a row.

My commute to and from the office was even more distressing. I was constantly pulling over to the side of the road: Intense pain in my lower abdomen made it nearly impossible for me to sit up straight and focus on driving. The pain typically worsened throughout the day. I would get home from work and try different strategies to "move" whatever was causing the pain. After numerous trips to the bathroom, I could only get relief by lying on my side in bed.

"Stress" was just not cutting it as the explanation for my pain. I was twenty-three and supposedly healthy, but I wasn't. Was I simply doomed to spend the rest of my life in digestive agony? Such a bleak conclusion was not acceptable. My gut instinct (pun intended) told me there was more to learn.

I began to search for answers in earnest, but all my doctors' appointments stuck to the same script. An identical examination, followed by an identical diagnosis:

"IBS."

"Irritable bowel syndrome."

"IBS…It's becoming quite common."

Over and over again, that's what I was told. But the only accurate part of the term "IBS," in my opinion, was the "BS." Possibly, this diagnosis was "quite common"—because the doctors were *quite commonly missing the cause*. No mention of a food allergy ever came up, despite my repeated indications that I felt the worst immediately after eating. The doctors refused to see the connection between what I was eating and how I was feeling.

After more fruitless examinations than I care to remember, I was completely fed up. I was also in unbelievable pain around the clock. At that point, I was willing to try absolutely anything to get answers. After undergoing a "recommended" sigmoidoscopy—a minimally invasive intestinal procedure that yielded no clear diagnosis—I began to feel even worse. None of the medication I was prescribed for my stomach seemed to help, and I was tired of relying on doctors for solutions that never seemed to come. One doctor actually put me on an antianxiety pill. The reason? One of the medication's side effects was that it numbed the stomach lining. The doctor had completely missed the mark.

That day set me, fuming, on a more determined search. There had to be a more direct means of treating whatever was going on with me. I refused to spend the rest of my life bouncing from doctor to doctor—or taking serious prescription drugs hoping for their side effects to kick in. If my own physicians were not helping me, I was going to get to the bottom of this mystery on my own.

From that day forward, I dove into research. I met with a holistic doctor in a neighboring state, who put me on a dairy-free, lactose-free, yeast-free program. Under his care, I went on a whole regimen of supplements and vitamins, and I lived off these special bars, which I was allowed to eat three times a day. I ate apricot seeds every day, as he told me they would help. The seeds were the most vile-tasting things I had ever tasted, but I kept on eating them in the hopes of feeling better. Even though they seemed to burn my tongue, I was willing to give them a shot. To my dismay, not even these extreme measures brought about any significant changes in my condition. Still, I resolved to do whatever it took. If that guy had told me to stand on my head for ten minutes every hour, I would gladly have done it for eleven.

As we were about to begin the phase of removing wheat from my diet, I applied to become a contestant on the reality show *Survivor: The Australian Outback*. Throughout the selection process, I hid my symptoms from the producers, saying nothing about the stomach pain that I was experiencing. As I went through extensive physical exams, I was amazed that no one could tell that the inside of my body was a complete disaster. I held back tears during one exam, which entailed the doctor pressing on my stomach. I held my breath as the doctor told me I was "good to go"…secretly counting the seconds until I could race to the bathroom.

Early the next morning, miraculously enough, I was picked as a contestant on *Survivor*, and so off I went, pain and all, into the Outback.

My Australian adventure was nothing short of life-altering. It was an incredibly rich, rewarding time—physically, mentally, and spiritually. Not surprisingly, it was the most physically grueling experience of my life. I was also given the most wonderful opportunity to investigate how my body works. Though exhausted on every level, I felt awakened. I learned how to live off the earth, to respect its boundaries, to work and bond with strangers, and to get by without any creature comforts. I also learned what mattered to me most, and what I relied on in extreme circumstances. One other remarkable thing happened to me Down Under, too: For the first time in about three years, I felt no pain in my stomach.

I remember thinking on multiple occasions, "Even though I haven't showered in thirty-nine days, I feel clean and pure." I was fairly certain that this sensation had nothing to do with my skin or hair or scent, and everything to do with my internal system. I was completely detoxified—without pain, without cramping or bloating, without any intestinal symptoms at all. I felt like I had before I had checked into the college infirmary so long ago. That person seemed to be nearly forgotten.

Shockingly, it took *starving* in the outback of Australia to feel like myself again. I remember joking that "I must be allergic to the United States." That was not the case.

I had lost about twenty pounds, but though my belly was empty, I left Australia full of answers. I left knowing that without God, I had nothing; that my family was the most incredible source of support; that I never again wanted to be away from Tim. I left knowing that for the past three years, my body had been fighting something that I was eating at home, and that if I didn't take it upon myself to figure out what that food was, no one else would do it for me.

Once I was back home, the scope of my quest narrowed.

Energized with the sense that I was on the trail of the culprit at last, and with a clean slate, I decided to reintroduce one item at a time back into my diet. But after thirty-nine days in near-starvation mode, I was absolutely ravenous, and I wasn't about to give up my favorite foods without a fight. Soon, despite my best intentions, I had returned to my pre-Australia diet, and the consequences were dire. After the relief of having had my gut repaired, now I was suddenly feeling worse than ever, spending day after day in my room, unable to get out of bed, except to race to the bathroom.

They say that every cloud has a silver lining, and this horrible time finally clued me in to the cause of my long illness. I noticed that the moment I ate a starchy food, all the symptoms returned, and with even more fury than before. I went on the Internet to research what this reaction might mean, and soon after thought I had discovered the cause: *Wheat!* Out it went from my diet.

There were some days when I didn't feel so bad. Still, every so often, I would get tripped up after eating sushi or teriyaki chicken, and I couldn't put my finger on what was making me sick. After more and more online research, I stumbled upon some information about gluten intolerance and celiac disease. In 2002, *five* years since the onset of my symptoms, I diagnosed myself with celiac disease, an autoimmune condition triggered by gluten, the protein found in everything from pasta to bread to cookies. The only known treatment for celiac disease—which can cause acute damage to the small intestine and the digestive system as a whole—is a lifelong gluten-free diet.

Since celiac disease seemed to cover each of the symptoms that had been plaguing me for so many years, I set about eliminating all wheat, then barley, oats, and rye—the main gluten-containing foods—from my diet. In the beginning, the road was rocky: There was so much I still had to learn about gluten, and finding desirable alternatives was not as easy as it is today. I also found myself repeatedly rebelling against my self-diagnosis, and bingeing on gluten-containing foods just to prove that I could have them if I wanted to. Despite these repeated slipups, I nevertheless persevered…And my body would soon thank me.

Even after this breakthrough, doctors resisted my self-diagnosis. Though I was convinced that I had celiac disease—and armed with plenty of specific examples to back up my claim—I still could not find a physician who would run the necessary diagnostic tests on me. Dismissing the theory that my diet could cure me, doctor after doctor kept on prescribing medications that did little more than mask my symptoms, if even that.

I began to wonder why so many doctors ignored my theory—and why I had to spend months learning about celiac disease on my own. There had to be a reason why such a common disease, which affects an estimated 1 out of every 100 to 200 people worldwide, was not on medical radar at all. The more I thought about it, the more I came to believe that there was no money in researching gluten intolerance, because there was no medication to treat it. No noise, no advertisement, no call to diagnose. Was this the result of some conspiracy? Neglect? Straight-up ignorance? Whatever the explanation, I had to struggle for eight long years before I found a physician who was willing to listen, willing to run proper tests, and willing to join me on the voyage that I'd been on since 1997.

Ironically, I had to travel all the way to Australia to gain real insights into what was hurting me in the United States, and when I moved to New York City, it was an Australian, Dr. Peter Green, the director of the Celiac Disease Center at Columbia University, who confirmed what I'd suspected for years. The moment he told me I had a disease—celiac disease—I enthusiastically thanked him. This reaction might seem a little bit odd, but I had been searching for a clear-cut diagnosis for almost a decade by then! I had consulted innumerable experts in the hopes of finding out what was wrong with me. For all those years I had waited in vain for an explanation that made sense. Dr. Green was the first doctor to look for the cause, not simply treat the symptoms. My gratitude to him is beyond measure.

Once Dr. Green confirmed that I had celiac disease, I became even more committed to what I called the G-free lifestyle. With Dr. Green's help, I deepened my knowledge of where gluten is found, and how I could most effectively avoid it. With the encouragement of my loved ones, I became more adept at shopping for and preparing delicious G-free alternatives to what had once been my favorite foods.

In no time at all, I found that living G-free wasn't so bad at all! In fact, I've never felt better in my life. I cannot imagine *ever* returning to eating gluten—even if I *didn't* have celiac disease. The G-free diet gives me the stamina and strength I need to manage my increasingly hectic life.

It turns out I have a lot of company! Apparently, I am not alone in benefiting from the G-free diet: According to the University of Chicago, 1 out of every 133 otherwise healthy adults in the United States has celiac disease—that's nearly 3 million of us.

But a gluten-free lifestyle can help countless others as well. People suffering from a wide range of diseases—from autism to osteoporosis, from diabetes to rheumatoid arthritis—can often benefit from this change in diet. Even people with no health issues have a great deal to gain by giving up gluten. The G-free diet can help with weight management. It can elevate your energy levels, improve your attention span, and speed up your digestion.

Whatever your motivation for going G-free—whether you have celiac disease or a gluten intolerance, or a basic desire to live a healthier, longer life—this book will help you achieve your goal. It's an all-inclusive, easy-to-read survival guide to living without gluten and *loving* it. I will define gluten in all its particulars, and teach you how to spot it in the unlikeliest places. I will also help you navigate social situations, and instruct you in the art of reading both food and beauty product labels. You will learn how to target gluten-free products, both at restaurants and your local supermarket, how to stay on your diet even in a foreign country, and even how to keep your kids G-free in the school cafeteria. By the end of this book, you will be equipped with all the information you need to get through the world without gluten. My guess is that you will only wish that you had done it sooner!

2

What Is Celiac Disease?

Celiac disease is a digestive disorder characterized by a toxic reaction to gluten, the protein found in certain grains. Celiac disease is hereditary, meaning it's in your gene pool; chronic, meaning it won't ever go away; and autoimmune, meaning it causes the body to attack itself.

It's important to remember that celiac disease is *not* a food allergy, and you can't pop pills to "cure" it. The only known treatment is a *gluten-free diet for life*, a subject we will explore in much more detail later.

If you have celiac disease (which is also known as celiac sprue, nontropical sprue, and gluten-sensitive enteropathy), gluten damages the tiny, hairlike villi lining your small intestine and prevents your body from absorbing the nutrients it depends on to survive. The nutritional deficiencies that result from this chronic malabsorption can lead to a staggering range of serious health problems.

While scientists once considered celiac disease an extremely rare

---

Celiac Disease on the Rise?

Celiac disease does seem to be affecting more people in recent years—and not simply because doctors are getting better at diagnosing it. "One possible explanation for the increase," said Dr. Andrew Weil, the director of the Integrative Medicine Program at the University of Arizona and the author of *Eight Weeks to Optimum Health* and *Healthy Aging*, "is that we've been breeding wheat for higher and higher gluten content, so there's been greater exposure to gluten. Another explanation is that the increase in incidences of celiac disease is one aspect of a general toxic overload in the world today."

---

childhood disease, they now know that it's one of the most common genetic conditions in the world. In fact, researchers believe celiac disease might affect as much as 1 percent of the population worldwide. In this country, roughly 3 million people, or 1 out of every 133 Americans, have the disease. A great many more people might have what's known as gluten sensitivity, which is a less severe reaction to gluten.

What makes these numbers even more alarming is that less than 5 percent of those who have celiac disease know it! In the United States, it takes an average of *nine to eleven years* to diagnose a celiac patient after the first onset of symptoms. Compare that to Europe, where diagnosis often takes place within a year of the first appearance of symptoms.

The diverse and deceptive symptoms of celiac disease make it exceptionally difficult to diagnose, but if you even *remotely* suspect that you might have this condition, waste no time in talking to your doctor about your concerns. Untreated celiac disease can take a severe toll on your health, leading to a number of complications including intestinal cancers, Type 1 diabetes, osteoporosis, miscarriage, and infertility.

The longer a person who has celiac disease consumes gluten, the more likely these conditions are to develop and worsen. Even if you are symptom-free, you are still not off the hook. (See Chapter 3 for more on this.) Getting tested for celiac disease could be one of the most important decisions you will ever make.

What Causes Celiac Disease? Who Gets It? Why?

All excellent questions—and ones that some of the most brilliant doctors and researchers in the world are still scrambling to answer! Our bodies work in mysterious ways, and the medical community still has a *lot* to learn about the causes and triggers of celiac disease. This is what we know, to date.

Who: While people of all ages, genders, and ethnicities can have celiac disease, it's more prevalent in certain populations, particularly in people of Northern European descent. (In Finland, celiac disease is so widespread that every McDonald's in the country offers gluten-free buns!)

Because celiac disease is genetic, the rates are much higher for people with celiac family members. If a first-degree relative—a parent, sibling, or child—has celiac disease, your chances of getting diagnosed are about 1 in 22. If a second-degree relative—an uncle, or cousin, or grandparent—is affected, your odds are roughly 1 in 39.

Why: To have celiac disease, you must carry the gene for it. We also know that people suffering from other autoimmune disorders—Type 1 diabetes, thyroid disease, Down syndrome, Sjögren's syndrome, ulcerative colitis, and many others—have higher incidences of celiac disease. Doctors believe that celiac disease can make people more susceptible to these conditions (with the exception of Down syndrome), even though those disorders are usually flagged first, while all too often the primary cause—celiac disease—goes unnoticed, undiagnosed, and untreated. This neglect only worsens the related autoimmune conditions in the long run.

When: A person can "come down with" celiac disease at any age, but doctors have identified several peak diagnostic periods. Many celiac patients are diagnosed in infancy, between the ages of nine and twelve months. Most likely, these diagnoses occur because parents pay such close attention to food and allergen introduction in their infants' menus. Other people with celiac disease do not show symptoms until decades later, generally in early adulthood.

Carrying the gene for celiac disease is not necessarily enough to activate the condition. Other factors play a role as well, some better understood than others. For full-blown celiac disease to develop, you must typically meet the following three criteria:

1. You carry the gene for celiac disease.
2. At the time of testing, your diet includes gluten. (Removing the gluten does not cure the disease, but it does erase most symptoms.)
3. You undergo some sort of physical or emotional trauma that activates or "switches on" the condition.

The first two are clear as day. How exactly do experts define Number 3? Well, they believe that many different events might qualify as "trauma": surgery, pregnancy, childbirth, a viral infection, a serious physical injury, or any sort of severe emotional stress.

I have no doubt that, in my case, the trigger was the bacterial intestinal infection I came down with in Belize during my sophomore year of college. That infection clicked on my celiac disease, and my system has never been the same since. The main problem was not my eventual diagnosis but the amount of time I spent searching for it—ten long years. Five years of improper nourishment, and of symptoms that ruled my days. Ten years I can never get back. Ten years that will affect the rest of my life.

Possible Symptoms

There are no "textbook" symptoms of celiac disease, which at least partially explains why it's so pervasively underdiagnosed. Celiac symptoms vary widely, and they aren't always gastrointestinal in nature. Some symptoms are constant; others are occasional. And as I mentioned earlier, some celiacs have no symptoms at all.

For these and other reasons, doctors frequently confuse celiac disease with other conditions like irritable bowel syndrome, acid reflux, Crohn's disease, intestinal infections, and chronic fatigue syndrome. (Celiac disease is a multisystem disorder, with symptoms that are just too wide-ranging to meet any tidy diagnostic checklist.)

Any of the following problems might be an indicator of celiac disease:

- Abdominal pain and discomfort
- Anemia and other deficiencies
- Constipation
- Delayed puberty
- Diarrhea
- Discolored teeth
- Distension
- Excessive weight loss (with a large appetite), or weight gain
- Fatigue
- Gas
- Headaches
- Joint or bone pain
- Loss of dental enamel, tooth discoloration
- Missed menstrual periods

- Muscle cramps
- Reproductive problems (infertility, multiple miscarriages)
- Skin rashes, itchiness
- Smelly stool
- Sores inside the mouth
- Stunted growth in children
- Tingling or numbness in legs
- Vitamin K deficiency

Patients might have other sensitivities as well, including lactose intolerance, an allergy to casein, or a peanut allergy. Chemical sensitivities are also common. Dermatitis herpetiformis (page 24) is a form of celiac disease that manifests itself in the skin, in persistent rashes and bumps that itch, redden, and/or peel.

Long-Term Conditions Resulting from Untreated Celiac Disease

If you don't absorb nutrients over a long period of time, it's only logical that you will develop a number of lasting health problems. Without the proper fuel, you cannot expect your body to stay strong and healthy. Untreated celiac disease has been linked with all of these health issues:

- Infertility, spontaneous miscarriages
- Intestinal cancers
- Iron deficiency anemia
- Folate, potassium, and vitamin B12 deficiencies
- Osteoporosis
- Rheumatoid arthritis
- Thyroid problems
- Fibromyalgia
- Type 1 diabetes

Doctors have also seen evidence that gluten sensitivity and celiac disease can potentially influence mood and behavior disorders like ADHD, depression, and bipolar disorder. Experts are currently studying the link between gluten and autism spectrum disorders, as there is strong evidence that removing gluten from the diet can vastly improve the condition.

Talking to Your Doctor

The medical community is a long shot away from where it needs to be when it comes to the diagnosis and treatment of celiac disease. Underdiagnosis and misdiagnosis continue to be huge problems, especially in this country.

My own story, I'm afraid, is all too typical of what other people experience: For years after diagnosing myself with celiac disease, I struggled to find a doctor who would listen to my theories. When I told doctors—and there were lots of them—that I thought I had celiac disease, they looked at me as if I were crazy, or speaking a foreign language. Why were all these well-recommended doctors just flat-out dismissive of a condition that I knew was common all across the globe?

The answer, according to Dr. Green, is that too many physicians in America just don't know enough about celiac disease. "The textbooks are out of date," he says. "There's not a lot of education about the disease, and there's very little research being published in medical journals on the subject—doctors just aren't taught about it in this country."

In Dr. Green's home country of Australia, he said, "Roughly thirty to forty percent of people with celiac disease are diagnosed—about the same as in Italy and Ireland. In this country, less than five percent of those who have celiac disease get diagnosed."

What's behind these terribly low diagnostic rates? "One of the reasons celiac disease is so grossly underdiagnosed in this country," says Dr. Green, "is that the pharmaceutical industry has such a major role in the direction of health care here. In many countries around the world, where there are national health plans, doctors are actively encouraged to diagnose celiac disease. In this country, the pharmaceutical industry provides eighty percent of the money for medical research. It also provides a lot of money for postgraduate education, and there just aren't any drug companies that are interested in researching celiac disease. There's basically no money in it—no drug company will provide funds for the research."

Simply put: Since there are no drugs to treat celiac disease, pharmaceutical companies stand to gain no profits from encouraging its diagnosis.

"It's a general problem in our culture," Dr. Weil said of these lopsided priorities, "and I think it's both that people don't have the information and motivation to take responsibility for their well-being, and that the system is economically locked into paying for interventions with drugs, not for lifestyle counseling. The whole system is dysfunctional. It's all one big knot, and I don't know where you begin to push. In general, we're so locked into using pharmaceuticals to treat everything that when we come across conditions that we can't treat with drugs, we tend to pay less attention to them."

Be Your Own Advocate

If you suffer from any of the health complaints listed on the previous pages and you suspect gluten might be the cause, make an appointment with your doctor immediately. When the day of your appointment comes, make sure you are armed with adequate information. Keep a careful log of your symptoms, ask detailed questions, and mention your concerns about celiac disease. Do not simply expect a doctor to stumble upon this diagnosis for you.

Getting an Accurate Diagnosis

It might require some perseverance on your part to get an accurate diagnosis. First off, you should seek out a physician who is willing to investigate a disease that no medication can cure. Because the standard battery of blood tests that doctors run does not check for gluten intolerance or celiac disease, you need to be very precise about requesting tests that will. According to Dr. Green, many people in the United States get proper diagnoses only after they specifically ask their doctors for these tests.

"Patients often tell me," he says, "that when they ask their doctors to run tests for celiac disease, the doctor will say that they couldn't possibly have it: 'You're too tall, you're too fat, you're black, you're Jewish, you're not Scandinavian.' Then the doctor calls back to say the patient has actually tested positive—surprise, surprise. That's the only reason a lot of patients are getting diagnosed, because they're insisting on these tests."

Step 1 to diagnosis: Celiac panel. A celiac panel is a blood test which is generally the first step in diagnosing celiac disease, although it cannot deliver a conclusive celiac diagnosis. What it *can* do is rule out celiac disease, or determine where you fall on the risk spectrum. It tests for the presence of these antibodies associated with celiac disease:

- Antiendomysial antibody (IgA EMA)
- Antigliadin antibody (AGA-IgA and AGA-IgG)
- Tissue transglutaminase (tTG-IgA and tTg-IgG)
- Total serum IgA

Step 2: Endoscopy and small tissue biopsy is the next step in diagnosing celiac disease. You should *only* go through this invasive procedure if the celiac panel has shown your risk level to be high. To perform this biopsy, doctors insert a tube down your throat, which they use to remove a tiny piece of tissue from your small intestine. They then examine this tissue sample to determine whether your villi are damaged.

You should also be aware that gluten must be present in your system for most of the endoscopy and biopsy to provide accurate results. If you've diagnosed yourself with celiac disease and have already given up gluten on your own, your doctor might not be able to assess the results properly—but this is not always a good reason for going back on gluten!

Some doctors may request that, for a conclusive diagnosis, you embark on what is known as a "gluten challenge," which entails, according to Dr. Green, "eating the equivalent of about four slices of bread a day for a few months." A gluten challenge might not be necessary if you have yet to give up gluten. In that case, just continue eating your regular diet before going through the tests.

Step 3: Genetic testing is recommended if both Steps 1 and 2 prove inconclusive, which sometimes does happen. Doctors can test for the presences of the specific HLA (human leukocyte antigen) genes associated with celiac disease (DQ2/DQ8). While scientists don't yet know the exact genes involved in celiac disease, they do know that you *must* have DQ2 and/or DQ8 to develop it.

I encourage you to request these tests if you have any reason to suspect that you might have celiac disease. A proper diagnosis will put you on a path of well-being and steer you toward health…It could even save your life.

Points to Remember

- Celiac disease is a chronic, hereditary, autoimmune digestive disorder characterized by a toxic reaction to gluten. It is not a food allergy.
- Gluten is a protein found in wheat, barley, rye, and contaminated oats.

- The only known treatment of celiac disease is a lifelong gluten-free diet.
- Not everyone with celiac disease exhibits gastrointestinal symptoms—or any symptoms at all.
- Developing celiac disease depends on multiple factors, including the ingestion of gluten and an individual's genetic makeup.
- Diagnosing celiac disease is a multistep process involving blood tests and a small intestine biopsy.
- Failure to treat celiac disease can lead to even more severe health problems over time.

Fortunately, a gluten-free diet can seriously reduce your susceptibility to all of the long-term health issues associated with celiac disease. Once you get a proper diagnosis, you can finally begin to take charge of your health again. You will feel like a new person in no time at all, and to get there, all you have to do is go G-free!

Conditions Associated with, and Complicated by, Celiac Disease

Under any circumstance, giving up gluten is a big deal. Undeniably, the gluten-free diet seemed overwhelming when I first embarked on it. However—after countless days spent curled up on the bathroom floor, groaning in agony—I was willing to try *anything* to reclaim my heath. Since then, I have never looked back.

Of course, not everyone with celiac disease displays the sort of in-your-face symptoms that I had. A person with undiagnosed celiac disease might not even suspect that migraines, irritability, and fatigue might all point to a larger systemic problem in the body.

Or who knows—you might have absolutely no symptoms at all. Say, for example, your sister just got diagnosed and encouraged you to get screened as well. When your test results came back positive, you were probably extremely confused, not to mention defiant. Bread does not make you sick; it gives you energy! You can scarf down half a pizza and run a marathon an hour later—so why should *you* of all people give up gluten?

In this instance, you might be tempted to dismiss your diagnosis as meaningless and move on with your life. While I certainly understand the impulse, I am here to tell you why that would be a big mistake. Having no gastrointestinal symptoms—or no symptoms at all—in no way immunizes you against the many long-term health problems associated with celiac disease.

Celiac disease is what's known as a multisymptomatic disorder, meaning it can damage multiple parts of your body in addition to (or even instead of) your digestive tract. If untreated, it can harm your liver, your brain, your bones, even your dental enamel. According to the University of Chicago Celiac Disease Program, there are a jaw-dropping 256 symptoms and health conditions associated with celiac disease. This staggering range of related conditions is one of the big reasons doctors have so much difficulty correctly identifying and diagnosing celiac disease, even in patients who have been suffering for years.

And what if you *haven't* been suffering—if you have what's known as "silent" celiac disease? I will admit: I have a deep aversion to glutenous foods, as they only remind me of the pain and discomfort associated with losing control of my health. When I come into contact with gluten, my body reacts with such violence that I have no difficulty rejecting certain foods and ingredients. People who are

Understanding Dermatitis Herpetiformis

In his book *Celiac Disease: A Hidden Epidemic*, Dr. Peter Green describes dermatitis herpetiformis as "celiac disease of the skin." In other words, dermatitis herpetiformis is a form of gluten intolerance that manifests itself in the skin, in a pervasive, severe itchiness and blistering, particularly around the elbows, knees, and buttocks. Like celiac disease, dermatitis herpetiformis is frequently misdiagnosed, often confused with eczema, psoriasis, or some other skin condition. Also like celiac disease, dermatitis herpetiformis has only one known treatment: a strict, gluten-free diet for life.

asymptomatic face the rather different challenge of turning away from food that does not feel like it's doing damage. Going off gluten when your tummy seems just fine is not easy.

It is important to consider the following: You may be having symptoms and not recognize them for what they are. But even if you have *no* symptoms (at least not now), gluten *will* take a toll on your health in the long run—and continuing to eat it may cost you your life.

Possible Complications of Untreated Celiac Disease

The key word in the above heading is "untreated." As with so many other symptoms of celiac disease, the gluten-free diet will go a long way toward protecting you against these and other associated problems. In many cases, removing gluten is all it takes to repair whatever's ailing you. How many other serious health problems put that much healing power in the hands of the patient?

MALNUTRITION

Chronic malnutrition is the most immediately obvious complication of untreated celiac disease. Damaged villi prevent nutrients from being properly absorbed into the bloodstream. This is due to the normally large surface area on a healthy intestine becoming inflamed and flat, with less area to absorb nutrients. So no matter how much you are eating, your body isn't getting the vitamins and minerals it needs to thrive. As a result, you might develop iron deficiency anemia, or lose your dental enamel (what's known as *permanent enamel hypoplasia*), or contract any number of even more serious health problems.

SHORT STATURE, DELAYED GROWTH OR PUBERTY

Children deprived of proper nutrition during critical developmental periods seldom grow as fast as their peers, and no wonder:

They simply don't have the fuel. A gluten-free diet can help compensate for these delays, but according to the National Institutes of Health, if a child with celiac disease isn't diagnosed in time, his growth might be permanently stunted. Delayed puberty is another common side effect of undiagnosed celiac disease in children.

OSTEOPOROSIS

If you are not absorbing calcium, vitamin D, and other essential nutrients over a long period of time, your bones might become weak and brittle, which could lead to osteoporosis and other skeletal problems, including recurrent fractures and osteopenia. Osteoporosis—which can cause pain and fractures of the spine, hip, and other bones—is a fairly common side effect of untreated celiac disease. In fact, roughly 75 percent of recently diagnosed celiacs have some degree of bone loss. Luckily, you *can* protect yourself against osteoporosis, even if you spent many years searching for the right diagnosis. Talk to your doctor about getting your bone density tested. Depending on the results, you might need to supplement your gluten-free diet with calcium, magnesium, and vitamin D. Exercise also really helps rebuild bone mass.

CANCER

According to *Celiac Disease: A Hidden Epidemic*, people with celiac disease are nine to thirty-four times more likely to develop a malignancy than the general population. Adenocarcinoma, a cancer of the small intestine, is one of the cancers that affect people with celiac disease at much higher rates than the rest of the population. Rates of non-Hodgkin's lymphoma, esophageal cancer, and melanoma are also much higher among people with celiac disease. But again, adherence to the gluten-free diet can make these alarming numbers drop precipitously.

REPRODUCTIVE ISSUES

Researchers are still struggling to understand all the reproductive issues associated with celiac disease in both men and women. Over the last thirty years, the medical community has come to accept that incidences of unexplained infertility and recurrent spontaneous abortions are higher for women with celiac disease—as much as *four times* higher, according to a recent study conducted at the Thomas Jefferson University Hospital in Philadelphia. Preliminary results of a study in Turin, Italy, have found the prevalence of celiac disease among women with unexplained infertility to range from 2.5 to 3.5 percent.

And according to the National Digestive Diseases Information Clearinghouse (NDDIC), mothers with untreated celiac disease are more likely to give birth to babies with neural tube defects (like spina bifida), since their bodies cannot properly absorb folates and other nutrients essential to the health of a fetus. Celiac mothers also frequently have smaller babies and breastfeed for shorter periods than other women. Other reproductive issues they might experience include delayed periods, menstrual irregularities, and premature menopause.

Untreated celiac disease can have a negative impact on male fertility as well: Men with celiac disease tend to have a reduced sperm count and lower levels of male sex hormones.

If you and your partner are having reproductive problems, both of you should consider getting screened for celiac disease. A gluten-free diet can reverse or greatly reduce the severity of most of these issues, and fairly quickly, too.

MISCARRIAGE

The link between undiagnosed celiac disease and higher than normal miscarriage rates is also one that doctors are struggling to understand. "We don't know why there's increased infertility, especially an increase in miscarriages," said Dr. Green, "but the association is there. It's just unclear what the mechanisms are." Women with celiac disease not on the gluten-free diet had a 17.8 percent rate of pregnancy loss, compared to 2.4 percent of celiac women who were on the diet. After just six months on the G-free diet, these women saw a 91.8 percent reduction in miscarriages, resulting in similar miscarriage rates as the rest of the population.

NEUROLOGICAL ISSUES

People with undiagnosed celiac disease might suffer from various neurological problems, including migraines, *primary ataxia* (extreme imbalance and lack of muscular coordination), epilepsy, and different *peripheral neuropathies* (a broad term to describe tingling and numbness in the hands, feet, and other bodily extremities). Untreated celiac disease could even lead to *paraplegia*, or paralysis of the limbs. The gluten-free diet, if implemented in time, can diminish or even resolve many of these serious neurological complications.

DEPRESSION AND OTHER PSYCHIATRIC ISSUES

There are many reasons celiac disease and depression go hand in hand. If you are constantly sick to your stomach, if you are always hungry but never getting any nutrients, how could you *not* be a bit downcast? Scientists have identified a link between poor nutrition—and low levels of vitamin B12 in particular—and depression. Vitamin B12 and other B vitamins play an essential role in producing the neurotransmitters responsible for regulating moods and other brain functions. If you are not absorbing these and other nutrients, both your body *and* your brain will start to misfire at some point.

In some patients, the celiac diagnosis does not entirely resolve these psychiatric issues. Professional counseling can be useful in helping people who have difficulty coping or complying with the limitations of a gluten-free diet.

Additionally, irritability, attention deficit/hyperactivity disorder (ADHD), and anxiety might also result from untreated celiac disease. One study showed that people with celiac disease have ADHD symptoms, but researchers do not yet know if the G-free diet can lessen these symptoms.

LIVER DISEASES AND DISORDERS

Primary biliary cirrhosis and autoimmune hepatitis, among other diseases and disorders that cause the liver to function improperly, might be related to celiac disease. While experts have yet to determine the precise mechanisms of this link, they do know that people with celiac disease have higher rates of liver abnormalities than other segments of the population.

Celiac Disease and Related Autoimmune Conditions

Celiac disease, you will recall, is an autoimmune disorder, meaning it causes the body to attack itself. Autoimmune disorders can have a domino-like effect in the body: If you have one autoimmune condition, you are more likely to have two, or even three. While roughly 3 percent of the general population has an autoimmune disorder, ten times as many people with celiac disease do—that amounts to nearly 30 percent. This statistic suggests that celiac disease could predispose patients to other autoimmune diseases. "Having celiac disease," said Dr. Green, "may cause people to get these other autoimmune conditions."

But as is so often the case, the risk factor sharply declines with early diagnosis and treatment. (The flip side is also true: The quantity—and severity—of associated autoimmune disorders increases the longer celiac disease goes untreated.) The overlapping nature of autoimmune disorders can make celiac disease even more difficult to detect. Often, patients will be diagnosed with the peripheral autoimmune disorders instead of—not in addition to—celiac disease.

If you have any of the following conditions, you might want to talk to your doctors about getting tested for celiac disease as well.

THYROID PROBLEMS

In my mid-twenties, before I had stumbled on my celiac disease self-diagnosis, I went through long periods of listlessness. My whole life, I'd been athletic and high-energy, and suddenly I was dozing off all the time—even at the gym! No lie: I was even having trouble keeping my eyes open while running on the treadmill. Once on the mat to do some abdominal work, I would feel my eyes flutter shut again. I simply *could not* stay awake. I also noticed a change in my once-sharp memory: Forgetting where I'd parked my car was just not something common. Important information was noticeably becoming hard to retrieve from my short-term memory.

I was eventually diagnosed with a mild thyroid problem, which turned out to be one of the most common autoimmune conditions associated with celiac disease. Leading a normal life can be difficult if your thyroid is out of whack, since the thyroid gland is the control center for all your hormones, moods, and energy levels.

Some people with celiac disease have autoimmune thyroid disorders, like hypothyroidism (also known as Hashimoto's disease), or a thyroid gland that does not produce enough thyroid hormone. On the opposite end of the spectrum is hyperthyroidism (also known as Graves' disease), or too much thyroid hormone, which can cause severe weight loss, accelerated heartbeat, and weakness, among other symptoms. In most cases, doctors can bring thyroid levels back to normal with carefully monitored medication. And for patients with celiac disease, "There are studies," Dr. Green said, "that show thyroid function actually became improved on a gluten-free diet."

Had I simply relied on the singled-out diagnosis of a thyroid problem, I would still be suffering.

TYPE 1 DIABETES

Diabetes is a disease characterized by an inability to produce adequate insulin, which aids our bodies in using and storing sugars. Unlike Type 2 (formerly known as adult-onset) diabetes, Type 1 diabetes—or insulin-dependent diabetes mellitus—is an autoimmune condition. Roughly 6 to 10 percent of the estimated 1 million Type 1 diabetics in this country today will also develop celiac disease.

Other Autoimmune Disorders

Fibromyalgia is something of a catchall diagnosis offered when doctors can find no other explanation for pervasive pain in the muscles and joints. Nine percent of patients eventually diagnosed with celiac disease have at one time also been diagnosed with fibromyalgia.

Rheumatoid arthritis is among the fastest-growing autoimmune disorders in the country, affecting an estimated 1 percent of the population. Rates of *juvenile idiopathic arthritis* (which used to be called juvenile rheumatoid arthritis) are also steeply on the rise. Both disorders are characterized by joint inflammation, pain, and stiffness, and both might have a connection to celiac disease. Between 1.5 and 6.6 percent of children with juvenile idiopathic arthritis also have celiac disease.

Sjögren's syndrome is a connective tissue disease that occurs when the body's moisture-producing glands cease to do their job. Sjögren's patients, most of whom are female, suffer from extreme dryness of the mouth, eyes, and other mucous membranes. Roughly 5 percent of people with Sjögren's and other connective tissue diseases also have celiac disease.

Addison's disease is an autoimmune disorder of the adrenal glands, which help regulate our stress response, as well as our metabolism, immune and cardiovascular systems, and sex hormones.

Aphthous stomatitis is characterized by recurrent canker sores on the inside of the mouth. A gluten-free diet can lead to a significant improvement of this condition.

Cardiomyopathy is the medical term for an inflamed heart muscle. Removing gluten from the diet can improve this serious cardiac condition in celiac patients.

The old saying "an ounce of prevention is worth a pound of cure" applies to many aspects of health maintenance, not least of all your diet. If you have celiac disease, understanding the long-term benefits of going G-free can change—and even save—your life.

Childhood Syndromes Associated with Celiac Disease

Children born with certain chromosomal anomalies—specifically, Down syndrome, Turner syndrome, and Williams syndrome—have noticeably high rates of celiac disease. If your child has one of these disorders, you should consider routinely testing for celiac disease as well, since roughly 12 percent of children with Down syndrome, and an estimated 3 percent of children with either Turner syndrome or Williams syndrome, also have celiac disease. Why the overlap? Doctors still don't have all the answers. Some experts speculate that children with chromosomal disorders are at a higher risk of developing autoimmune disorders as a result of a general metabolic imbalance.

Gluten

KNOW THINE ENEMY

> GLUTEN: A yellowish-gray, powdery mixture of plant proteins
> occurring in cereal grains such as wheat, rye, barley....The gluten
> in flour makes it ideal for baking because the chainlike protein
> molecules of the gluten trap carbon dioxide and expand with it
> as it is heated. Gluten is also used as an adhesive and in making
> seasonings, especially monosodium glutamate (MSG).
> —*The American Heritage Science Dictionary*

Gluten is a protein found in wheat, barley, rye, contaminated oats (meaning they were grown, harvested, or processed in a gluten-containing facility), and a multitude of other products—as its word origin suggests, it acts as the "glue" that holds these foods together. Gluten is that sticky, binding substance that gives breads and pastas their elasticity and texture.

As you might expect, breads and other everyday foods like pizza, cookies, muffins, and bagels contain gluten, but so do a number of other items that may really surprise you. Because gluten is an all-purpose stabilizer and thickener, manufacturers add it to a wide range of consumer products. Medications, marinades, condiments, coffees, packaged spices, postage stamp adhesive, envelope seals, lipsticks, hairsprays, and even your daily multivitamin can all contain gluten as well.

If you cannot tolerate gluten, you should right away start familiarizing yourself with what exactly gluten is, and where it's found. Once you are armed with the correct knowledge, you can take the necessary steps to get the gluten out of your life. If you don't have a health issue related to gluten but still want to clean up your diet, you might take a more moderate approach to deglutening your diet. In that case, you might want to start by simply reducing, not all-out eliminating, gluten. Replacing your breakfast cereal with a G-free version and having your sandwich on G-free instead of white bread are simple ways to make those changes. Still, whether you go G-free in some or all aspects of your life, you should first understand what exactly gluten is, and where it's found.

Naturally Gluten-Free Foods

Before I get into what you *can't* eat, let's focus on everything you *can* feast on and enjoy whenever you want. All of the following in their pure form contain no gluten whatsoever:

- Lots of tasty, healthful grains, including:
    Quinoa
    Buckwheat
    Corn
    Millet
    And many, many more!!
- Fruits
- Vegetables
- Meat (untreated, unsliced)
- Chicken
- Fish
- Nuts
- Seeds
- Eggs
- Vanilla and vanilla extract in their pure form
- Spices in their pure form

Where Gluten Is Found

Gluten is an incredibly sneaky substance, hidden in the unlikeliest places. Let's start, though, with the most obvious sources of gluten: grain-based products made from wheat, barley, rye, and contaminated oats. All these common grains, especially wheat, have numerous derivatives and aliases. If you are new to the G-free lifestyle, keep the names of these wheat and barley derivatives with you on your next trip to the grocery store.

Off-Limits Grains

WHEAT

Wheat is an ancient food, a staple of much of the world's food supply for almost 10,000 years. It is the second-most popular cereal in the world, more common even than rice. Only maize (corn) is produced and consumed in greater quantities worldwide. Different cultures have processed wheat in an endless variety of ways—leavened it into breads, powdered it into flours, fermented it into alcohols. All of the following foods contain wheat (and therefore gluten) and should be avoided on the G-free diet:

- Bran: Bran is the fiber-rich outer layer of the wheat grain. A by-product of the milling process, bran is often used to enrich cereals and muffins.
- Bulgur: Bulgur is a dried, crushed, and debranned form of wheat that's popular in the Middle East. It's the main ingredient in tabouli salad.
- Couscous: Couscous is a spherical, semolina-based pasta that's consumed all over Northern Africa. It's often served in a meat or vegetable stew.

- Durum: Durum, also known as macaroni wheat, is the toughest wheat—its name comes from the Latin word for "hard." Also known as Abyssinian hard wheat (*Triticum durum abyssinicum*) and durum wheat (*Triticum durum*).
- Einkorn: Einkorn is a wild species of wheat that is easier to grow than other species of wheat. It is used to make bulgur, and for animal feed. Also known as *Triticum monococcum* and wild einkorn (*Triticum boeotictim*).
- Emmer: Emmer is used in breads, soups, and pastas. It's popular in Switzerland and Italy. Also known as farro, wild emmer (*Triticum dicoccoides*), or just *Triticum dicoccon*.
- Farina: Farina, a type of semolina, is the key ingredient in Cream of Wheat and other warm wheat-based cereals. Also known as farina graham.
- Farro: *See* Emmer.
- Graham flour: Graham flour is a whole-wheat flour used in graham crackers and piecrusts.
- Kamut: Kamut is a hard wheat similar in texture to durum.
- Matzo meal/flour: Matzo is made of flour and water. During Passover, Jews eat this unleavened flatbread.
- Orzo: Orzo is the Italian word for "barley." This tiny pasta resembles rice but is actually made out of semolina. (*See* Semolina.)
- Panko: Panko is a Japanese breadcrumb made from crustless bread.
- Seitan: Seitan, also known as "gluten meat," is a wheat-based alternative to tofu, used as a meat substitute in vegetarian dishes throughout Asia and increasingly in this country as well.
- Semolina: Semolina is a form of wheat before it has been ground into flour. Hard (durum) semolina is the main ingredient in couscous and many pastas. Soft-wheat semolina, or farina, is used in breakfast cereals and desserts. Also known as durum semolina, semolina triticum, and matzo semolina.

- Spelt: Spelt, or small spelt, is a popular type of hard wheat that has been grown in Europe for centuries. It has a higher protein content and is considered less allergenic than other forms of wheat.
- Udon: Udon is a type of thick wheat noodle that is often served in Japanese soups.

RYE

Rye—the key ingredient in rye flours, rye breads (like pumpernickel), rye beers, and some whiskies and vodkas—is closely related to wheat. Rye has a lower gluten content and a higher fiber content than wheat.

BARLEY

Half of the barley produced in this country is used as animal feed. When fermented, barley is used to make malt, a key component in the production of many beers and distilled alcohols. Coffee substitutes and instant coffees also frequently contain barley. If you see any of these words on a label, the food is likely to contain barley:

- Barley grass
- Barley *Hordeum vulgare*
- Barley malt
- Barley groats
- Pearl barley
- Malt and malt flavoring: These two additives are often but not always made from barley.
- Malt vinegar: Malt vinegar is almost always made from barley. Many other types of vinegar are safe. (See page 81 for a list.)
- Caramel color: Caramel color is another additive that can be made from barley malt. Check the label or call the manufacturer, as some caramel colorings are safe.

Wheat by Any Other Name...

Wheat comes in many different guises and answers to many different names. I suggest studying this list and familiarizing yourself with all the different names for wheat. If you see any of these terms on a list of ingredients, you can be sure that the food is *not* G-free.

Abyssinian hard (*Triticum durum abyssinicum*)

Club wheat (*Triticum aestivum* subspecies *compactum*)

Common wheat (*Triticum aestivum*)

Fu (dried wheat gluten)

Hard wheat

Hydrolyzed wheat gluten

Hydrolyzed wheat protein

Hydrolyzed wheat protein PG-propyl silanetriol

Hydrolyzed wheat starch

Hydroxypropyltrimonium hydrolyzed wheat protein

Macha wheat (*Triticum aestivum*)

Oriental wheat (*Triticum turanicum*)

Persian wheat (*Triticum carthlicum*)

Polish wheat (*Triticum polonicum*)

Poulard wheat (*Triticum turgidum*)

Shot wheat (*Triticum aestivum*)

Sprouted wheat or barley

Stearyldimoniumhydroxypropyl hydrolyzed wheat protein

Timopheevi wheat (*Triticum timopheevii*)

Triticale X triticosecale

Triticum vulgare (wheat) flour lipids

Triticum vulgare (wheat) germ extract

Triticum vulgare (wheat) germ oil

Vavilovi wheat (*Triticum aestivum*)

Wheat amino acids

Wheat (*Triticum vulgare*) bran extract

Wheat *Durum triticum*

Wheat germ extract

Wheat germ glycerides

Wheat germ oil

Wheat germamidopropyldimonium hydroxypropyl hydrolyzed wheat protein

Wheat grass (can contain seeds)

Wheat nuts

Wheat protein

Wheat *Triticum aestivum*

Wheat *Triticum monococcum*

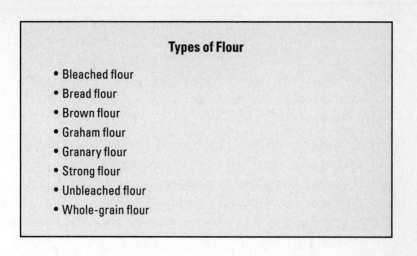

Types of Flour

- Bleached flour
- Bread flour
- Brown flour
- Graham flour
- Granary flour
- Strong flour
- Unbleached flour
- Whole-grain flour

TRITICALE

Triticale is a hybrid of wheat (Latin name: *Triticum*) and rye (Latin: *Secale*) developed in the late nineteenth century. Grown in areas where wheat is difficult to cultivate, this synthetic grain is mostly used in animal feed.

Questionable Starches

OATS

Oats remain a subject of great debate in the G-free community. While oats don't contain gluten, they are often grown or processed alongside wheat, so the risk of cross-contamination (see page 47) is fairly large. "By far the majority of people with celiac disease tolerate oats," says Dr. Green. "There are some very well-described cases of people who got the same intestinal lesion with oats, but that's an exceptional case." But, he adds, "Most oats are in fact contaminated and there are some gluten-free oats that can be used. But we advise people to eat gluten-free oats if they can get them. If people experience symptoms from eating contaminated oats, it's probably just because they're eating more fiber." Before consuming any oat product, investigate the brand and speak with your physician.

DEXTRIN

Dextrin refers to a category of polysaccharides made from starch. Dextrin can be produced from corn, potato, arrowroot, rice, tapioca, or wheat. While most U.S. manufacturers of dextrin use corn, imported dextrin is often made from wheat, so you shouldn't buy a dextrin-containing product until you've double-checked its source. Dextrimaltose is made from barley.

Hidden Sources of Gluten

When you swear off gluten, you will quickly learn that a standard loaf of bread is off-limits, but unfortunately, the distinction between G-free and G-full foods is not always this clear-cut. The G-free diet requires you to examine just about every food before putting it in your mouth.

The following list of products might contain hidden sources of gluten:

FOODS

Bacon bits and other imitation bacon products: Unless the package indicates otherwise, many imitation bacon products contain gluten. Hormel's Real Bacon Bits are gluten-free.

Beer: While you can find plenty of delicious G-free beers these days (see page 120), most traditional beers are made from barley, rye, and other gluten-containing grains.

Blue cheese: The mold that gives blue cheese its characteristic color usually originates on old bread, so I would stay away.

Brown rice syrup: Rice on its own is safe, but brown rice syrup is made from a combination of rice and barley malt.

Cereals: Most traditional cereals have a high gluten content. Unless a cereal is made *exclusively* from the G-free grains listed on pages 81–86, you should avoid it.

Coffees, flavored and instant: Avoid flavored and instant coffees unless you're assured they're G-free, and avoid sharing your coffeemaker with them as well. Decaf coffee can also contain gluten, so check that one, too.

Communion wafers: Many Catholic communities have already worked out G-free communion solutions for their celiac members. Ener-G Foods sells G-free communion wafers (www.ener-g.com).

Croutons: Croutons are made from dried, toasted bread. If you see any on your salad, send the whole plate back.

Dairy substitutes: Avoid dairy substitutes unless you are certain they're gluten-free. Vance's Dari Free (www.vancesfoods.com) is a potato-based milk substitute.

Deli meats: I only buy deli meats that say "gluten-free" on the label, as many have added gluten. Sausages, hot dogs, salami, and self-basting turkeys are even more likely to contain gluten. For more information, please see pages 88 and 220.

Fried foods: French fries, chicken nuggets, and other deep-fried foods might all be contaminated with gluten. Make sure that there is no gluten in the batter of any fried food that you order, and also that your food has not shared a deep fryer with any glutenous food, as cross-contamination can occur.

Gravies: Gravies are often thickened with gluten-containing products, so always eat your food dry unless you're assured that the gravy is 100 percent G-free.

Hydrolyzed vegetable protein (HVP) and hydrolyzed plant protein (HPP): HVP and HPP are used in many fake meats. If these are made from wheat, they are unsafe. If made from soy, they are safe. "Under the FDA, if they come from wheat, the source must be put in parentheses on the label," said Dr. Green. But he still recommends caution, since barley as a source would *not* necessarily be indicated on the label.

Imitation seafood: The imitation crab in California rolls might contain fillers made from wheat starch. Always check.

Licorice: Pure licorice is G-free, but most commercial licorice candies have added gluten. It depends on the brand, so be sure to read the label carefully.

Marinades: Stay away from all premade marinades such as teriyaki sauce. Almost all restaurant marinades have some gluten content.

Salad dressings: Many restaurants and food manufacturers add gluten to thicken salad dressings.

Seasonings and spices: In their pure form, seasonings and spices are gluten-free. But watch out for spices that contain added declumping agents, as these often contain gluten. If you don't see an ingredient list on the bottle, call the company and inquire about gluten and fillers. The term "ground spices" might indicate the presence of gluten, so be on guard against that one as well.

Soy sauce: Some soy sauces are gluten-free, but you can't bet on it. I recommend bringing your own G-free soy sauce along to Asian restaurants.

Soup bases: Commercial bouillon cubes and chicken, beef, and vegetable stocks often have added gluten. Do not buy any of these without reading the label, and do not order soup in restaurants without asking about the soup base.

OTHER POTENTIALLY GLUTEN-CONTAINING ITEMS THAT MAY SHOCK YOU!

Beauty products: I will be exploring this subject in more detail in Chapter 14, but in the meantime, you should know that many lipsticks, lip glosses, skin moisturizers, hairsprays, and other everyday beauty products might contain gluten, often in the form of wheat germ oil or hydrolyzed wheat protein.

Stamp and envelope adhesive: The adhesive used in stamp and envelope adhesive is likely to contain gluten, so play it safe by using sticker stamps and moistening envelope flaps with a sponge.

Play-Doh: While experts don't yet know if gluten can be absorbed in the skin, the gluten content of Play-Doh is a problem because children often place their hands—and their toys—directly into their mouths.

Prescription drugs and over-the-counter medications: Some prescription drugs contain gluten-based filler ingredients, also known as *excipients* or *inert ingredients*, added to the active drug. You have to be really careful because most pharmaceutical companies don't list which excipients they've used either on the bottle or in the package insert. You might just see the word "starch," with no information about where the starch comes from.

While some starch-based excipients are made from corn, potato, and tapioca, others are wheat-based. Therefore, proceed with caution. Talk to your doctor *and* your pharmacist about the gluten content of the medications—both prescription and OTC—that you take. If you still have questions, call the manufacturer.

Unfortunately, you have to go through this process every time you get a refill, for several reasons: Pharmaceutical companies frequently change the inactive ingredients without warning, and generic drugs often have different excipients than the brand-name version of the same drug. For more information, check out www .glutenfreedrugs.com. You will find lists of medications (Advil, Aleve, Visine A, Pepto-Bismol, Nyquil, and many more) that manufacturers list as gluten-free.

Vitamins and supplements: Decoding the additives in vitamins and nutritional supplements has gotten a lot easier over the last few years. Under the Food Allergen Labeling and Consumer Protection Act of 2004, nutritional supplements must be labeled if they contain wheat (barley and rye are not used). Still, you should always talk to your pharmacist about the gluten content of different vitamin brands, or ask your doctor to recommend a safe, G-free supplement. If you are still not convinced that the vitamins you are taking are safe, get on the phone with the manufacturer right away. (For tips on making these calls, see page 75.)

Rule of Thumb

If you see the word "starch" on the list of a medication's inactive ingredients, don't take that drug until you have identified the source of that starch.

Label Detective: Recognizing Glutenous Terms

As you start to navigate the world without gluten, you will need to become an expert label reader—and I am here to teach you this essential skill. You will soon have all the tools you need to read (and even better, to understand!) the labels of a wide range of consumer products, all in a matter of seconds. You will also get in the useful habit of keeping tabs on your favorite items to make sure their ingredients haven't changed when you were not looking.

The good news is that deciphering labels gets easier every day. Under the Food Allergen Labeling and Consumer Protection Act of 2004, food manufacturers must clearly label all products that contain any of the eight most common food allergens: wheat, milk, eggs, fish, shellfish, tree nuts, peanuts, and soybeans. But while this new labeling protocol is a huge improvement—and a boon to celiacs everywhere—you should still be on your guard, because as we know, a food could be wheat-free and still contain gluten. (Corn flakes, for example, contain no wheat, but they often do contain barley malt.) The FDA is in the process of developing universal *gluten*-free labeling for foods and medications.

Another warning: Foods under the supervision of the U.S. Department of Agriculture instead of the FDA—meats, coffee, dairy products—are held to a different set of rules altogether. "If it's USDA," said Dr. Green, "they don't have to declare what it's from, or whether or not it contains wheat, so it can be confusing. If the food is from the USDA, you have to get that information directly from the manufacturers."

In Chapter 7, I will walk you through the step-by-step process that I rely on to determine the gluten content of a product. For now, I just want to familiarize you with the red flags that may signal the potential presence of gluten in a product.

- Additives: Way too vague for my comfort zone. You need to find out exactly what those additives are.

Reminder

Since the term "gluten" also includes barley and rye, do *not* make the common mistake of confusing the term "wheat-free" with "gluten-free." A food can contain no wheat and still have a high gluten content. What's more, the term "gluten-free" is unregulated in this country, so there are no agreed-upon amounts of "safe" gluten levels. There is also no standard international definition of "gluten-free."

- Artificial color: The words "artificial color" or just "coloring" on a label might indicate the presence of gluten. Unless I know exactly where that coloring comes from, I am not going to eat it.
- Brewer's yeast: While brewer's yeast generally contains gluten, all other types of yeast are considered safe.
- Emulsifiers: Emulsifiers or "emulsifying agents" might be synonymous with gluten.
- Filler: Filled with what? Anytime you see such a vague word on a label, be very, very wary.
- Germ: Germ is usually a synonym for wheat, so watch out!
- Glucose syrup: Glucose syrup is generally made from corn, potatoes, or wheat. Check the source before consuming.
- Grain alcohol: The American Dietetic Association believes that the distillation process removes the gluten content of these grains, but I still tend to avoid these products.
- Groats: The word "groats" can refer to any dehusked grain, but it is usually applied to oat products. You must make sure that any oats you eat have been processed in a G-free facility.
- Hydrogenated oils: Hydrogenated soybean oil does *not* contain gluten.
- Malt: While malt *could* be made from corn, it's usually made

from barley. Malt extract, malt syrup, malt flour, and malt vinegar are all no-nos. Other vinegars are G-free.

- "Modified food starch": In the United States, the single word "starch" by itself on a food label must come from a corn source, but "modified food starch" or "modified starch" could refer to any number of substances. If the source is wheat, the label must indicate that, per the Food Allergen Labeling and Consumer Protection Act. Still, that same rule does not apply to barley or rye, which could also be sources. Unless the word "modified" is defined here, you should play it safe and assume that it might contain gluten. The terms "vegetable starch" and "edible starch" are also questionable. Always check before consuming.

- "Natural flavor" or "flavors": If you see these vague terms on a label, run the other way! "Smoke flavoring" is also usually a bad sign.

- Softener: Gluten is often added to a product to make it softer and more elastic, so if you see this word on a food label without any further detail, either call the company or stay far away.

Understanding Cross-Contamination: The Basics

If you're just trying to clean up your diet and cut back on gluten, then you are probably safe steering clear of the most obvious G-full foods like pasta and bread. On the other hand, if you have celiac disease, a wheat allergy, or any other health problem associated with gluten consumption, even the smallest amount of gluten can hurt you. Going gluten-free means going gluten-free *all the way*. So not only must you avoid bagels and pizza and other obvious suspects, you must also turn away any foods that have even come into contact with these substances. This is the phenomenon known as cross-contamination.

This is where things can get really tricky. Cross-contamination occurs when a food that does not itself contain any allergens touches a food that *does* contain allergens. Cross-contamination can take place at any stage: If a G-free corn chip is processed on the same conveyor belt with a wheat- or flour-containing substance, then that chip has been cross-contaminated. If oats are grown, milled, processed, or stored alongside wheat, then those oats are cross-contaminated. If you drain G-free pasta in a mesh colander that has recently been used for G-full pasta, then that pasta has been cross-contaminated. If you slice carrots with the same knife that you used to slice bread, then those carrots have been cross-contaminated. It's these small, seemingly harmless exposures that will get you every time.

When you go G-free, you have to start asking endless questions, not just about the content of your food, but about a million little details surrounding its preparation. Were your eggs flipped with a gluten-contaminated spatula? Did that ice cream scoop touch a sugar cone? Did someone dust that cake pan with flour before filling it with G-free batter? Did that chicken share a grill with a glutenous marinade?

If you are as sensitive to gluten as I am, your stomach will soon answer those questions for you, though the actual source of the contamination will not always be clear. You will be left wondering what made you feel so awful. It won't be the wheat crackers because you no longer eat them. But could it be that the same knife that you used to spread dip on your G-free cracker was also used on the wheat-containing ones? You knew not to have the ice cream cone, but could your dessert have been scooped with the same scooper that went into the cookie dough ice cream? You become like a detective on *CSI*: You are always tracing your steps back.

Cross-contamination is a subtle, often invisible process, and it's 99 percent of the difficulty of remaining G-free. Which is not to say that it's impossible! There are lots of simple measures you can take to reduce your risk of eating cross-contaminated food.

How Much Gluten Can Hurt You?

Exactly how much gluten would it take to trigger symptoms?

"A slice of bread has about two and a half grams of gluten," explains Dr. Green. "Most people with celiac disease have an inflammatory reaction and symptoms with one hundred milligrams," or *about one twenty-fifth of a slice*, which is much less than a single bite. "Very few get symptoms or inflammation with ten milligrams. There's a case report of a woman in Italy who had the diagnosis and didn't get better and they traced it to the fact that she was having a corner of a communion wafer a day and that was calculated out to be one milligram of gluten. So there are different sensitivities." Still, if you think about how even minuscule amounts can cause a reaction, you understand why cross-contamination can be such a problem.

AVOIDING CROSS-CONTAMINATION

- Oversee food preparation like a hawk.
- Ask tons of questions.
- Read all labels carefully.
- Educate your friends and family members about how cross-contamination works. Teach them about all the little ways that gluten can get into your body. Talk to waiters, too, and anyone else involved in the preparation of your food. The more people know, the safer you will be!
- Keep separate utensils and maintain their integrity. For more information on this, see Chapter 6.

These long lists of G-full products and warnings about cross-contamination can be intimidating at first glance, and I am sure you are wondering right now if you will ever eat again. The answer is a resounding *yes*. There is a world of G-free foods out there just waiting for you, and you might be surprised by how delicious they are!

Points to Remember

- Gluten is the protein found in wheat, barley, rye, and some oats.
- Many unlikely foods and products, including shampoo and vitamins, might actually contain gluten. (There is some debate whether gluten in shampoo and body products can hurt you, but—as I discuss in detail in Chapter 14, "Gorgeously G-Free"—I always like to play it safe.)
- Mastering the fine art of reading labels takes some practice, but will be well worth it in the long run. Familiarizing yourself with all the different synonyms for gluten is a good place to start.
- "Wheat-free" does not mean the same thing as "gluten-free." A product could contain no wheat flour, but be filled with rye or barley.
- Avoiding cross-contamination is the biggest challenge of the G-free lifestyle, but it can be done.

5

Your G-Free Road Map

You might be giving up gluten because you've been sick for a long time, and your recent diagnosis with celiac disease has come as a big relief. You might be giving it up kicking and screaming, because although you've had no symptoms, your doctor says you have no choice. Maybe you are going G-free because your pediatrician has suggested a gluten-free, casein-free dietary intervention for your autistic child, a subject I'll be discussing in detail in Chapter 16. Or perhaps you simply want to lose a few pounds before swimsuit season! If this is your goal, even removing just a little gluten from your diet can be an effective weight-loss tool.

Whatever your motivation may be, adapting to a new diet—and by extension, a new lifestyle—is fraught with challenges. My own transition to G-free living was anything but swift. When I first read about celiac disease (*years* before I got an official diagnosis), I thought that going "gluten-free" sounded completely fanatical. Despite matching every single one of my symptoms with those of someone with celiac disease, I was *not* about to let some random

Web site dictate what I could and couldn't eat for the rest of my life. My instinctive response was not compliance, but full-on rebellion. I thought to myself: Oh, *really*? You think I can't eat gluten? Oh, yes, I can: Just watch me now.

Instead of giving up gluten right on the spot, I decided to prove that not only could I eat gluten, I could eat it in champion quantities. I went out and bought a family-size container of Oreo Double Stuff cookies, then proceeded to consume the entire bag in one night. Needless to say, I nearly passed out from pain and nausea, and was soon crouched on the kitchen floor hating my headstrong nature. Then again, I rationalized, who *wouldn't* be sick after consuming an entire bag of Double Stuffs?

Even after that, I continued bingeing on the very foods that the celiac Web sites were telling me were off-limits. Maybe I was trying to ambush myself to the point where I could no longer question my self-diagnosis. Having just a little wheat wasn't clear-cut enough for me. I was determined to go all out, to prove my allergy beyond any doubt.

Eventually, I was convinced: After every gluten binge, I would be on my side for a week, racked by unbelievable abdominal pain. Still I kept on sabotaging myself. By the end of the third month, I could no longer deny that gluten, and nothing else, had been the culprit all along.

That self-destructive phase has long since passed, and looking back, I cannot *believe* that I ever played Russian roulette with my body like that. Though I love the smell of fresh bread coming out of a bakery's doors on a Sunday morning in New York City, I am no longer even remotely tempted to taste it. The memory of the pain is still prominent in my mind, the damage to my intestine was done, and I *never* want to feel that way again. Between my loving family—including my two little ones (and another on the way!), whose days I am determined to make full and fun—and my vigorous work schedule, I simply don't have the option to pass out in bed for three or four days at a stretch. Would I slack off a little if not for those factors? Maybe. As it is, with my family and my work on my heart and mind, remaining G-free is clearly the only option for my future.

I have been G-free for seven years. I've never had more energy in my life. My memory has improved. I no longer experience muscle or joint pain. My overall alertness is much better, too—and that's after having two kids! I no longer feel as if my body is fighting itself. Not only does food satisfy me, but I'm able to work out and train harder because I'm no longer in a state of internal warfare. Once you set out on this path, I am confident that you will thank yourself every single day for making this lifestyle change. You can decide to go on the G-free diet today. Making the transition will take a little time, as you will be not only transforming your kitchen shelves, but also revamping your entire relationship with food. These adjustments don't happen overnight, and some days will be better than others, so go easy on yourself! The following mental reminders have worked to keep me G-free and happy, and I hope they can help you do the same.

Tomorrow Is the Best Remedy for a Terrible Today

Sometimes after I would accidentally have gluten, I would feel defeated and depressed. I would think to myself: "Well, I might as well have more!" Instead, on a bad day, I would call my mom. She would tell me, "Today is over. The good news is that tomorrow, you have a fresh start." A good message to take to heart, and to remember that regardless of a new diet or another big change in your life, or your reasons for being on that diet, everyone has occasional lapses—think of them as hiccups—especially early on.

Trust me: Even if your body responds miraculously well to the G-free diet, there will still be days when you do not feel that great. Every once in a while, you will crave foods with gluten. Or you will be at a wedding, and after accidentally eating a sauce that contains gluten, you think to yourself, like I do: Well, if I had the sauce, then I might as well have the pizza. And if I had the pizza, I might as well have the garlic bread…and on and on.

These slipups happen to everyone—do not waste time beating yourself up about it. The important thing is to get back on track ASAP. And you can! Your body is resilient and forgiving, so just focus your energies on getting back to where you need to be.

Your Body Is a Genius!

So you have gone on a major gluten bender, and hit the reset button to start over. Now you just need to put a little faith in your body—it was built to weather the most challenging storm. "The body has enormous capacity for regeneration," says Dr. Andrew Weil, "and the digestive tract especially is very good at that. I think if you stop putting in the irritants, and you do things that help the digestive tract heal, there's every reason to believe you can heal all the damage."

The truth is that if you have been G-free for a good chunk of time, the first few days after "getting glutened" will be really tough. Speaking for myself, if I do meet up with gluten, I feel intense pain, fatigue, loss of concentration, moodiness…followed by an insane craving for more of the same. In my imagination, I can only com-

---

Defensive Strategy 1

Stock up on foods that resemble glutenous foods, but that are G-free. For example, when you get into that crazed craving mode, rip into a box of Pamela's cookies, Xochitl chips, or Glutino crackers. You are still going to feel overstuffed, and regret your binge-fest. But at least the damage you've done is short-term, and not long-term.

Defensive Strategy 2:
Sweat It Out to Get It Out!

To speed up the detox process, I will hit the elliptical machine or the road regardless of how terrible I feel, just to break a sweat. "I think that strategy is as emotional as it is physical," said Pat Manocchia, the owner of La Palestra Center for Preventative Medicine in New York City. "I think that's an effort on your part to control it. You feel like it's not beating you up, that you've got a say in this. I don't know if I would recommend [strenuous exercise], but what I can say is that from a purely physiological standpoint, the body only heals with circulation. And by exercising, you're increasing your circulatory system. You're allowing it to bring healing nutrients to the places that need to heal and take away the toxins."

For gentler ways of sweating out the gluten, you could also try a steam bath, or a really hot bath with Epsom salt. The faster you can get that gluten out of your body, the sooner you will feel like yourself again. Every body is unique, of course, so talk to your doctor about creating a detox strategy that will work for you.

pare this reaction to that of an addict who has just ingested a forbidden substance: Even the most minuscule morsel of gluten will send me spiraling for the next three or four days. Though my stomach will be killing me, I must battle my desire to continue poisoning myself with more gluten.

However difficult (or even excruciating!) it might be at first, you have to get back into the saddle as soon as possible. "The day after eating gluten," Dr. Weil says, "you have to make a real effort not to ingest any. And remind yourself that your body *will* bounce back—it's very resilient. You should also try to drink plenty of water and make sure that you're moving your bowels. All of those measures are really important."

Whatever digestive crime you have committed, do not let your brain stop your body from starting afresh. It will take a few days to feel sane and G-free again, but you *will* get there.

First the Breakup, Then the Makeup

If you are among the 12 million Americans who have at least one food allergy, or one of the 30 million with food intolerances, you probably know what it means to have a complicated relationship with food. Struggling against your body at every mealtime can really take the joy out of eating.

Over the course of my twenties, I went from loving food to completely fearing every single thing I put in my mouth. When I first went G-free, I approached food as a fuel—period, end of story. I remember several years ago a woman at a dinner party turning to me and saying, "Isn't this meal exceptional?"

"We'll see tomorrow," I thought to myself. In my mind, food was exceptional if it didn't hurt me. It was exceptional if I could leave the dinner table in one piece, if I did not have to go home with the seat fully reclined, waiting to pull over for a rest stop, if I did not spend the next three days curled up in the fetal position.

Despite some really great experiences with chefs who tried hard to make things taste good for me, I still had a long way to go in terms of repairing my relationship with food. It wasn't until I was pregnant and eating for the benefit of my child that I made a real effort to take pleasure in eating again. I went on a mission to find and make G-free foods that tasted good and made me excited about eating again. I discovered that, with a little know-how, the G-free diet can be as varied and delicious as anybody else's.

Getting to a better place with food is absolutely possible. Living without gluten does *not* mean giving up your passion for food—you will get it back tenfold!

Knowledge Is Your Armor

At first, the doctor's order to "give up gluten" might send you spinning. The same day that her then two-and-a-half-year-old daughter, Katie, was diagnosed with celiac disease, Kathy Burger headed to the health food store to restock her kitchen.

"I was the mom who was going to conquer the world," she said. "I remember standing in that aisle and reading about everything Katie couldn't eat. It was overwhelming, so I just picked up a whole bunch of random things—I didn't know what else to do! I brought them home, and when Katie tasted one, she was ready to throw up…because the food was that horrible. And my husband tasted it and tried to fake enthusiasm, but he thought it was awful, too. It was hard. That's the worst part in the beginning, the feeling of being so overwhelmed and thinking, 'What am I going to feed my child?'"

I met Kathy when she was an audience member on *The View*. When she told me that her young daughter had just been diagnosed with celiac disease, I felt an instant connection with her and what she was going through. We have kept in touch ever since.

Kathy's experience is probably familiar to a lot of people who have had to give up any major food group for medical reasons. Upon first getting diagnosed with celiac disease, many people do not even know what gluten *is*, much less where it's found.

One of my primary motivations for writing this book was to provide you with all the information you need to confidently navigate the world without gluten. The more you learn, the less constrained you will feel when it comes to choosing foods that nourish you *and* taste good. As you familiarize yourself with everything you *can* eat, you will start to feel more in control of your diet, and more comfortable around food in general. Without fear of the unknown hovering over every meal, you can finally let yourself enjoy food again. Conquering this unknown requires equipping yourself with the essential information.

Studying up on gluten will not only make eating fun again, but will also protect you from the pitfalls of a too-restricted diet. Knowing all you can about gluten and the better alternatives out there will grant you the freedom to eat as diverse and interesting an assortment of foods as anyone else.

Replace, Not Remove

This is *crucial*: Throughout this book, as I discuss various aspects of the G-free diet, I am never talking about solely *eliminating* gluten. It is about *replacing* gluten with healthier, high-quality alternatives. This is not a weight-loss trend that calls for the removal of breads and most other carbs. The G-free diet, as you will see, is about *substituting*, with a food that will heal you for a food that your body is not meant to have. For example, instead of having more wheat-based food, why not try exchanging it with rice?

Misunderstanding this point will undermine the benefits of the G-free diet, and undercut the potential that you have to improve your health. You might be saying, "I could *never* live without my sandwich at lunch every day." Don't worry—there is no reason for you to give up that sandwich! You will just be replacing your usual wheat bread with gluten-free bread that will satisfy your hunger and strengthen your immune system. "If I am trying to get someone off gluten," says Ashley Koff (www.ashleykoffapproved.com), the go-to celebrity dietitian and author of *Recipes for IBS*, who customizes expert solutions for optimal health, "and that person is used to having a cookie every day, well, that's fine. Maybe three months down the line I'll say, let's try not having that cookie. Let's try replacing it with fruits and nuts, or we could even start making that cookie at home. But initially, we can certainly replace that cookie with a gluten-free cookie that is very similar to what they were used to having every day."

"If you take a food away from someone," she went on, "they are more likely to become obsessed with that food. So instead of removing pasta from a person's diet altogether, I will suggest replacing it with a gluten-free quinoa or rice pasta. You can't just say, 'Okay, no more pasta. Have a salad instead.' You have to make gradual shifts."

This principle is key: Diets fail a person the second he or she feels deprived. "Removing without replacing" might help you lose weight in the short term, but this is neither healthy nor sustainable. If you are taking something out of your diet that contains elements your body needs, like the fiber in wheat, you need to seek out nutritious substitutions—especially since the G-free diet is about a long-term, lifestyle change. If you indeed have celiac disease, then you have gone without necessary nutrients for far too long. Now is the time to begin the healing process, and to give your system the nutrition it has been lacking.

A Dose of Perspective Goes a Long Way

Getting diagnosed with celiac disease is both a blessing and a curse. The curse is obvious: You have a chronic autoimmune disease, and you can no longer eat what may have been some of your favorite foods. Not now, and not twenty years from now. Not ever again, without serious consequences. You also can no longer casually swipe any old food off the shelf and dig in. For the rest of your life, you are going to have to ask questions, to read labels, to discuss and be aware of every item of food that you eat.

As you begin making adjustments, you might understandably overlook the silver lining here, which is that you have the unique ability to make yourself feel 100 percent better.

I would bet that most victims of disease would give anything to hear that they could be healed with food. In your case, you will not have to rely on an infantry of doctors, heavy-duty medications, and invasive surgeries. The great thing about celiac disease is that all you have to do is remove certain foods from your diet, and replace them with ones that are ten times better for you.

Don't get me wrong—I am not saying that giving up gluten is easy, but when faced with the option of prolonged discomfort or a G-free muffin, it sure seems less daunting. So the next time you gaze at that bag of pretzels and start feeling sorry for yourself, take a step back. Yes, you have a disease, but you also know *exactly* how to control it—you have been given an instruction manual on how not to be sick! Will the beginning of the G-free diet be a cakewalk? (Pun intended!) No, probably not. Is better health within reach the moment you start eating this way? Absolutely!

Just say it: "I am going G-free."

Great! Now, let's get you there...

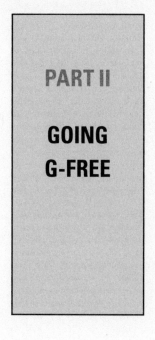

PART II

GOING
G-FREE

6

What's Mine Is Yours (Well, Sort Of!)

THE (MODIFIED) G-FREE KITCHEN

Whether you have celiac disease or any serious gluten intolerance, you should waste no time in refitting your kitchen into a safe place to prepare and enjoy gluten-free foods. Remember, cross-contamination is the unseen enemy of the G-free, and the smallest details *do* matter.

There are two different lines of attack you can take when G-freeing your kitchen. There's the all-or-nothing strict No Gluten Allowed approach, and then there's what I call the modified or compromised G-free kitchen, which harmoniously houses both G-free and gluten-containing foods.

Every once in a while, I think that if I could start from scratch, I would go the white-gloves route: install a gluten alarm on the front door, and permit no gluten inside my house under any circumstances. However, with the ratio of celiac to nonceliac being one to three in my family, I have chosen a compromise instead. Our kitchen, therefore, falls into the modified category, accommodating both the G-free and the G-devotees. (If you are just G-freeing your life gradually, then you can adopt an even more relaxed approach than the one that works for us.)

Sound like a complicated balancing act? Trust me, it isn't. With a little organization (and half-serious threats!), you can easily stay G-free at home without depriving your loved ones of their favorite glutenous pastas and pizzas. Stick to a few simple guidelines, and you will remain safely G-free.

Tip 1: It Ain't Easy Being Clean

WASH YOUR HANDS FREQUENTLY

I am glad there's no hidden camera in my kitchen, or I might just be mistaken for the most neurotic human being in the history of the universe. That's because I wash my hands *all the time*, especially after coming into contact with any gluten-containing products. After making my daughter a sandwich on wheat bread, I wash my hands. After I cut up her chicken finger, I wash my hands. After I make her dessert, I wash my hands. Get the basic idea?

GET THOSE DISHES AS CLEAN AS YOUR HANDS!

There's absolutely no reason to go out and buy your own G-free silverware and dishes, but you *do* need to make certain that everything is washed thoroughly after each use. A dishwasher can be a great tool for keeping your silverware and dishes clean, sterilized, and 100 percent G-free. So far, relying on our dishwasher has worked fine for me: I've never had any cross-contamination problems with our silverware or dishes.

DITTO FOR ALL COUNTERS AND COOKING SURFACES

This tip is just a logical extension of the last two. If you are preparing glutenous substances in your kitchen, you should wash down your counters and cooking ranges more regularly than seems alto-gether sane. Do *not* let any gluten-containing crumbs sneak onto your plate.

CLEAN OUT YOUR SILVERWARE DRAWER

While silverware drawers tend to be major crumb collectors, yours should be spic-and-span—and entirely G-free. It does not matter how clean that spoon is when you take it out of the dishwasher. If it comes into contact with invisible breadcrumbs in the silverware drawer, then your next G-free meal might very well leave you groaning.

Tip 2: Think Strategically

KEEP YOUR TOASTER AWAY FROM YOUR SILVERWARE DRAWER

Location, location, location: If at all possible, avoid positioning your toaster directly over your silverware drawer. Why? Because toasters produce crumbs, and crumbs like to lodge in those little compart-ments where you store your knives and forks. So if your silverware drawer is right underneath your toaster, it really does not matter how vigilant your family members are: They'll still be inadvertently sweeping crumbs over *your* forks and spoons every time they butter their morning bagel. So just play it safe by positioning your toaster as far away from your silverware drawer as you can.

LABEL YOUR G-FREE GROCERIES, ESPECIALLY IN THE REFRIGERATOR

Labeling your special G-free foods is absolutely essential if you are sharing your kitchen with gluten. Before sticking my G-free foods in the fridge, I mark them with little labels with my name on them. (The effect can be pretty bizarre sometimes: it reminds

Toaster Times Two?

Some people with celiac disease recommend having two toasters in the kitchen: one for gluten, one entirely G-free. Unfortunately, our all too typical (i.e., small and cramped) New York City kitchen just can't accommodate that setup. I'd rather eat food cold than figure out a place for a second toaster!

So while I do share the toaster oven with the rest of my gluten-loving family, I would never under any circumstances stick my food directly onto the crumb-encrusted rack—just looking at it gives me stomach pain!

Modified Kitchen Tip: I always put my G-free foods on foil before sticking them into the toaster oven. (You need a toaster *oven* to do this—you should never share a vertical slotted toaster with gluten.) If the bottom of my G-free bread does not get toasted enough, then I just flip it over and hope for the best.

me of a communal college refrigerator, with battling roommates staking out their private culinary territory!) Of course, everyone is always welcome to my food, but my little labels often seem to function like police tape: You *can* cross that line, but proceed with caution!

CARVE OUT A G-FREE SECTION OF YOUR PANTRY

Whenever possible, I stock my G-free foods—pastas, dry packaged goods, and dinner ingredients—along with my family's. But I also have my own little section in our pantry, where I store my Pirate's Booty and Pamela's cookies and other favorite snacks. I just find it's more convenient for me: When a craving seizes me, I don't have to weed through everyone else's food before striking gold. I just go straight for the bottom-left-hand corner and dig in!

KEEP YOUR FOODS AWAY FROM GLUTEN-CONTAINING BREAD

Bread is easy to keep separate since most G-free breads and waffles have to be kept in the freezer. But try not to keep your food near loaves of gluten-containing bread.

Tip 3: Double Up on Certain Items—and Label Accordingly

DOUBLE-STOCK CERTAIN FOODS, AND SEPARATE YOUR SPREADS

Double-stock any food that you spread across a piece of bread: cream cheese, butter, peanut butter, honey, jams, jellies—anything that a knife would go in. Even if my family and I eat the exact same brand of peanut butter, I always buy two identical containers. After all, it's often not the actual mustard that's the problem, but the mustard's potential contact with gluten.

LABEL YOUR G-FREE FOOD

It's important to label your spreads, too, so that family members know not to stick their crumb-encrusted knives in there. As with everything else in our kitchen, the entire family is welcome to all of

---

Compromised Kitchen Tip: Spray It On!

If you are steering clear of potentially contaminated sticks of butter (and you should be!), try spraying on olive oil whenever you need a nonstick surface. You can buy cans with olive oil already in them (Bertolli makes one), or you can buy a spray bottle and keep refilling it with olive oil whenever you run out. I do both!

my foods, but I have a strict policy against double-dipping—I will have your head if I see any breadcrumbs in my peanut butter or jelly!

HAVE G-FREE VERSIONS OF SELECT KITCHEN EQUIPMENT

You don't need to invest in a new set of pots and pans, but I do really recommend keeping two versions of several basic items on hand—one for gluten-containing products, and one reserved exclusively for the G-free. Here are my priorities:

Spatulas: Take a long hard look at that spatula you use to flip your eggs. Peer closely at all the nooks and crevices. Let's have an honest moment: Do those little stripes in the plastic ever *really* get clean, or is there always that bit of gunk that lingers even after multiple dishwasher cycles? Exactly what I thought. That's why I have my own spatula reserved exclusively for G-free foods.

Wooden spoons: The same goes for wooden stirring spoons. Any utensil made out of a porous material like wood can be dangerous, so buy some brand-new stirring spoons and designate them G-free. As always, make sure to label them clearly. Apply this better-safe-than-sorry rule to any utensils that seem difficult to clean. Keeping a few extra spoons around does not take up any room, and the peace of mind is well worth the added effort.

Baking sheets: The baking sheet I use for making cookies with my daughter—or for heating up gluten-containing pizzas—never, ever touches my G-free foods. As with the spatulas and spoons, I just worry that there's always some residue that never quite comes out. Trust me, you will enjoy your G-free cakes and cookies much more when you are certain that they have been made on their own sheets.

Cutting boards: Keep two cutting boards: one for bread, and one for everything else. I never use the bread cutting board for vegetables, meat, or anything else G-free. Even if your cutting board is straight out of the dishwasher, in my mind, the risk of cross-contamination is still too high.

Colander: Have a strainer to use exclusively for glutenous pasta—and *never* drain G-free food with it. The starch in pastas creates a filmy residue that's almost impossible to scrub out entirely, especially on mesh strainers. So err on the side of caution and use your own G-free colander.

Egg pan: Consider buying your own omelet pan, or any sort of small pan reserved exclusively for your eggs. When making eggs, rethink using the butter from the regular family supply, as it's most likely contaminated.

By making these simple and inexpensive changes, you have successfully deglutened your kitchen. Now it's time to get cooking!

Action Checklist

- Be ultrahygienic in the presence of food, regularly washing your hands, plates, utensils, and all cooking surfaces.
- Teach your family not to double-dip a knife that has touched gluten.
- Double-stock certain foods and cooks' tools, labeling the G-free version so no one gets confused.
- Designate a special section of your pantry a G-free zone.

So What *Can* I Eat?

G-FREE GROCERY SHOPPING

Living without gluten is one of the absolute paramount choices you can make to protect your health and improve your overall quality of life. But remember what I said earlier: Removing items from your diet without replacing them is a dangerous game. The G-free diet is *not* about deprivation. On the contrary, it's about feeding your body healthful, delicious foods that will sustain, nurture, and heal you. G-free or not, you need a varied, well-rounded diet in order to thrive.

We are all human. I still hit that cupboard late at night and root around for food, exactly as I did in my gluten-eating days. After my husband and I put the kids to bed, I want a good snack as much as any other parent. You, too, will probably be seized by cravings on a regular basis. The last thing you want to happen is to open the cupboard after a long day, and find absolutely nothing there you can eat. I have been there, and it is no fun. You will be faced with a choice at this vulnerable moment: either to go unsatisfied, or to binge on an unsafe food that will land your stomach in turmoil for the next three days. To avoid such digestive mishaps, load your kitchen with foods that can satisfy those cravings without making you sick.

Whether you have celiac disease, are trying to lose weight, or you just want to feel more energized by giving your body the best possible nutrition, you should always stock your refrigerator and pantry with foods that you *can* have so that you won't be tempted to eat foods that you cannot. Arm yourself with an interesting variety of staples and snacks: plenty of fresh fruits and veggies; some commercially prepackaged G-free frozen dinners; G-free chips, nuts, seeds, and crackers; candy or ice cream—whatever your comfort foods are in the salty, sweet, crunchy, hot, and cold categories, make certain they are there. Sometimes, I imagine that I am having G-free guests over and shop to stock up on new goodies. It is a fantastic strategy to try some new items, as well as to make certain you have a shelf *packed* with treats for that late-night chow-fest!

Now…let's go shopping!

Ingredient Detective: Determining the Gluten Content of a Food

Finding your way around a grocery store is one of the first skills you need to master in your early days of living without gluten. It can be both confusing and intimidating to go shopping immediately after making the switch to being G-free—but once mastered, shopping can also be an incredibly empowering activity. The more familiar you are with all the gluten-free options out there, the less you will miss the foods that were making you sick.

Some foods (ordinary bagels, muffins, and so on) are obviously banned on the gluten-free diet. Other foods (fish, fruits, veggies, nuts) naturally contain zero gluten; these are described in detail on page 34. But many, many other foods fall into a more mysterious middle category, forcing you to ask: Do they or do they not contain gluten?

Arriving at satisfactory answers will require dedication on your part. Early on, you may find yourself examining the label of each and every food you buy every time you go to the supermarket. And that's not all. What happens if, even after staring at the fine print for a good ten minutes, you are still not sure whether a food contains gluten? I will walk you through my methods for determining which foods are safe and which foods are anything but.

AT HOME

Twenty minutes of online research could save you twenty dollars or more—to say nothing of the cost of ingesting a food that is not meant to be in your body. So before you grab a cart, grab your computer!

Step 1: Research manufacturers' Web sites. Before you do anything else, visit the manufacturers' Web sites of foods you usually shop for to see if they contain gluten.

At the same time, you can visit the Frequently Asked Questions page of the company Web site to see if the manufacturers have already addressed the product's gluten content.

If you find that your favorite foods do contain gluten, research some smart alternatives on the Web. This way, even before you get to the grocery store, your "scavenger hunt" will be easier because you already know certain items are safe. Once you get there, with your list of G-free options, you can have fun loading the cart!

Step 2: Follow up your research on Google. If, after poring over a company's Web site, you still have unanswered questions about a food, Google is a good second line of defense. Try typing the brand/product name and "gluten" in the search bar to see what pops up. Do be warned, though, that not all Web sites are created equal, and some "information" on the Internet is unresearched and too sub-jective to be trusted. Opinions do not count as facts, so be certain that whatever you are reading is substantiated.

Step 3: Visit some celiac forums. You might also hit your favorite online celiac forums to see if other consumers have wondered about the very food you are itching to try. Blogs like www.glutenfreegirl .com, celiac disease forums (www.glutenfreeforum.com and www .forums.glutenfree.com), and general Web sites like www.celiac .com all have reliable information on the gluten content of specific products.

The beauty of the Internet is that you can visit all these Web sites simultaneously. Browse them all, contact companies when you can, and begin building your own go-to-G-free grocery cart! And remem-ber: For your first time shopping, do not panic…It is a process.

AT THE STORE

Your investigation picks up the moment you walk through the automatic doors. At first, this experience might seem like going to a Yankees game in a Red Sox T-shirt: You will absolutely feel out of place. But don't worry! Before too long, you will feel as comfortable and in command as you always did when browsing the aisles.

Step 1: Take a deep breath. There are two (perfectly understand-able) knee-jerk responses you should try to avoid:

- Do not walk out. I have done that. But you have to eat *some-thing*, and a grocery store is the best place to start remaking your diet. Just enjoy an adventure that will turn out to be more fun than scary.
- Do not rebel. In your panic, you might decide to buy sev-eral superpacks of whole-wheat bagels, cookies, and wheat crackers—I have done that, too.

Where to go?

Where you shop can be as important as what you buy when you get there. For best results, mix it up: Buy your basics at a conventional supermarket, then fill in the blanks at smaller health food stores and online bulk grocers. As long as you prep ahead of time and carry a list of safe brands with you, you will find the basics you need at a regular grocery store. For G-free flours and other harder-to-find items, you will have to hit the health food store. Once you hit on products you like, you can stock up at online stores, like the Gluten-Free Grocer (www.glutenfreegrocer.com). Refer to "Resources" for a complete list of recommended outlets.

Neither reaction was productive, or much fun for that matter. Take a breath, take out your list, and take that store by storm. Sooner than you think, shopping will become not about what you cannot have, but what you *can* have. Trust me.

Step 2: Scrutinize the label—every last word. Good work: You have gotten over the first and most difficult hurdle. Now that you have that cart rolling, keep your eyes peeled for foods that seem fairly natural, meaning they look like they came from the earth. Study the label carefully, going over every last ingredient and looking out for words like "modified" and "hydrogenated." Suspiciously vague terms like "natural flavors" or just straight-up "flavors" are also usually a sign that you should put the product on the shelf, or on your "Web-vestigate" list to refer to when you get back home. *Unless you can confirm the source with the companies, I would avoid foods containing these ingredients.*

Once you're at the store, you probably do not want to limit yourself only to the foods you researched in advance. Before making any purchases, though, you should always study the label carefully. If you don't see any dead-giveaway code words for "gluten" on the

---

Label Lingo

Remember: "Wheat-free" and "gluten-free" are not necessarily synonyms—a food could contain no wheat but have barley, rye, or oats. And a food does not have to be labeled "gluten-free" to contain no gluten. Lots of foods are naturally G-free. If you do your detective work in advance, you won't be left wondering which ones are which.

---

label (refer to page 38 for a list) and decide the product is safe to buy, still get back on the Internet when you return home.

BACK AT HOME

Step 1: Check again online. Before you tear into food you purchased but are unsure about, learn more about it. First you can go back online.

Step 2: Call the company directly. Still not sure? Now your only line of action is to call the company directly. Become a straight-to-the-source consumer. (I call up companies *all the time*: When I was pregnant, I was always craving a new food, and was on the phone with a different business nearly every day.)

In most cases, you will find customer service representatives eager and willing to help you out—most of them chose their careers because they love talking with and assisting people. One of my very favorite calls happened when I was pregnant and called up M&M's. The most wonderful woman talked me through every variety of M&M's. She also told me that callers asked her about gluten "all the time." Not only did I open up a bag of M&M's immediately after getting off the phone, but I felt a sense of fellowship with other people who had been in the exact same position before me!

Many food manufacturers will even have an on-site nutritionist or allergen specialist to consult with you. Additionally, the companies have their own stake in providing you with accurate information: After all, they don't want a lawsuit on their hands. So don't be shy about asking questions, and don't hang up until you are sure you have the most up-to-date information.

Step 3: Call back periodically. Yes, it sounds like a hassle, but "better safe than sorry" is your new mantra, and following up with companies can pay off. Call back every so often to make sure any

---

If Your Tummy Cries "Treason," There *Has* to Be a Reason!

I recently fell in love with a brand of corn chips that I thought was completely G-free. I had double- and triple-checked all the ingredients, and everything seemed safe. In all honesty, I loved the chips so much that part of me was subconsciously avoiding calling the manufacturer for fear of bad news. But finally, after about the eighth time of feeling awful after ripping through a bag, I forced myself to call the company's 1-800 number.

Sure enough, though the ingredients were gluten-free, the chips were passing down the same production line as a product made completely of wheat. My intention was to calmly explain that this processing information should also be put on the label, as people with celiac disease can become sick if they ingest gluten without knowing it. Instead, I was feeling so betrayed that I blurted out: "Do you know I have had the runs for four days, because you fail to mention that on the bag?"

Bottom line (no pun intended): Your stomach and system are the best judge. If a food that you think is completely safe is making you sick, there may be gluten lurking. Whatever you do, do *not* forget to ask about manufacturing and processing sites, and if your food of choice goes down the same conveyor belt as gluten-containing foods. A food doesn't have to have gluten on its list of ingredients to be cross-contaminated!

once-questionable foods are still gluten-free. Companies frequently change their manufacturing sites or acquire a new brand without altering their product labels. If you are buying chips, cereal, or any other grain-based food from a major company, you want to check that the product is not only G-free, but processed in G-free facilities as well. A corn chip could be riding down a clean conveyor belt one week, and dusted with wheat cracker residue the next. Even if you've been G-free for years, you may want to do these follow-ups on a regular basis.

Last but not least…Step 4: Bon appétit! If, after completing all these steps, you are confident that your new purchase is G-free, then the only thing left to do is rip into it and chow down! You will enjoy the food that much more if you know it's not going to hurt you.

Yes, it sounds like a lot of work, but this process is a big step toward putting you in control of your health. And trust me, if you've suffered through years of unexplained illnesses, it can feel pretty exhilarating to sit in the driver's seat for a change.

The Starch Situation

If you are like me, the word "starch" on a label might cause a little panic button to go off. But don't worry, because by U.S. law, the single word "starch" on a list of a food's ingredients *must* come from corn. The term "modified food starch" is much less clearly defined, however, so you need to call the company (page 75) to verify how exactly the "modification" took place, and with the help of which additives. Also note that this law only applies to food and not to prescription drugs and over-the-counter medications (see pages 43–44). The word "starch" on a list of a drug's inactive ingredients could refer to any number of sources.

Naturally G-Free Foods

The foods on the outer aisles of the supermarket should be the foundation of your diet—of any diet, really, with or without the gluten. Basic, natural foods that have kept humans going since long before the invention of sliced bread...

But first, one general guideline: You will notice in the next few pages that I use the word "pure" over and over again. That's no accident. I really can't emphasize enough the importance of selecting foods as close to nature as possible, in every sense of the term. In the produce section, that means fruits and vegetables that haven't been sliced, diced, mixed, or otherwise altered. In the meat section, that means chicken, meat, and seafood that have not been premarinated, precooked, presliced, or combined with other ingredients. There's no such thing as too pure at the grocery store!

Fruits: There's no more satisfying snack than a piece of fresh, delicious fruit. Always have apples, oranges, bananas, berries, or whatever else is in season in your kitchen. Canned and frozen fruits, in their own juices, are usually safe, since fruits aren't usually processed in wheat-containing facilities (unlike, say, oats, which almost always are). But do check the label to make sure no unspecified preservatives or emulsifiers have been added—that's where you could run into problems. As for fruits that have been cut and packaged in the store, be on alert: You just don't know what that knife was doing before it cut into that watermelon or

---

Rule of Thumb

The closer a food is to its natural state, the more likely it is to be gluten-free. When manufacturers process foods, they are often adding those hidden glutens that get us in trouble! In the G-free universe, simple often translates to safe.

pineapple. Though I have to admit, the cut watermelon still always ends up in my basket!

Vegetables: It's easy to get your greens on a gluten-free diet! Vegetables in their pure form are always 100 percent G-free, but do be wary of presliced veggies and store-mixed salads, which might be prepared with gluten-contaminated utensils.

Meats: Lamb, pork chops, ground beef, steaks, and other red meats are naturally gluten-free. Study the labels carefully to make sure no cross-contamination has occurred. I'd steer clear of bacon and sausages not specifically labeled gluten-free, as they might contain gluten fillers. Veggie burgers and other vegetarian meat alternatives are also risky, as most are made from wheat-based seitan. Telling the butcher that you have a serious allergy and asking him to put on a fresh pair of gloves is always a good strategy.

Poultry: Chicken, turkey, duck, quail, and other birds are gluten-free. But again, make sure the poultry you buy has been packaged and stored out of gluten's reach. And ask lots of questions before bringing home any preseasoned turkey or chicken burgers. To be on the safe side, you should always marinate everything yourself.

Fish and seafood: Tuna, salmon, trout, cod, shrimp, scallops, anchovies, sardines, clams, mussels, lobsters, oysters—you can eat these and many other creatures of the sea, as long as they haven't come into contact with gluten on their trip from the ocean to your plate. Avoid any imitation seafood products—like the fake crab-meat used in vegetarian sushi—because they are often made with glutenous fillers. Before buying any canned fish products, make absolutely sure that they are gluten-free.

Nuts: I'd think twice about prebagged trail mixes, but in their pure form, nuts—pistachios, macadamias, walnuts, cashews, pine nuts, and so on—make an ideal low-sugar, high-protein snack. Nuts can also be converted into multipurpose oils and butters.

Seeds: Pumpkin seeds, sunflower seeds, sesame seeds, and poppy seeds are great for snacking and for adding zest to other foods. Some seeds, like amaranth and quinoa, also make delicious, satisfying main courses. Chia seeds are also a wonderful source of essential fatty acids.

Beans, legumes, and tofu: High-fiber, low-glycemic-index beans and legumes make wonderful building blocks for any diet. Whether dried or canned, they are almost always gluten-free. Just buy them plain, and add your own flavorings at home. Tofu, a soybean by-product, is another versatile everyday food that's low in fat and high in protein.

Fresh eggs and pure egg substitutes: Eggs contain no gluten, but do your homework when shopping for multi-ingredient egg substitutes. Some brands might have a form of gluten on the ingredient list.

Vanilla and vanilla extract: As long as the vanilla is sold without any added colorings or flavors, it's safe. Always check with the manufacturer to be certain.

Spices: Beware the anticlumping agents added to many commercial herbs and seasonings (including those used at restaurants)—they almost always contain gluten. Stick to spices in their pure form. Check with the manufacturer to make absolutely certain that they contain no gluten. I would also recommend cleaning out your spice rack and starting over, since contaminated spices are one of the main routes of gluten exposure.

Popcorn: Popcorn is made from corn, and in its pure form contains no gluten.

Chocolate: Pure chocolate and cocoa contain no gluten. Lots of big-name chocolate bars are also gluten-free—I provide a list later in this chapter (see pages 91–92).

Dairy products: Milk, cream cheese, cottage cheese, and other dairy products are gluten-free in their pure form. For more on cheeses, see page 88.

Oils and butters: Most common cooking oils—olive, soy, safflower, grape seed, sunflower, corn, canola, cottonseed, coconut, and hydrogenated soy—are gluten-free. Butter is G-free, too, as long as you keep it away from crumb-contaminated knives! Ditto for margarines, creams, pure mayonnaises, and nut butters.

Vinegar: By U.S. law, balsamic, apple cider, and wine vinegars are made from apples and are gluten-free. But not all vinegars get the G-free stamp of approval: Grain vinegar may come from wheat, and malt vinegar is almost always made from barley. Most other vinegars in their pure form are safe.

Sweeteners: In their pure form, common sweeteners like sugar, honey, and maple syrup are gluten-free.

G-FREE GRAINS AND FLOURS

For me, the chance to discover these amazing grains—many of which I'd never even heard of before—remains one of the greatest thrills of going G-free. I am still learning about new grains all the time, and experimenting with different ways to prepare and enjoy them. Most importantly, my energy level is better than ever, as my new grains deliver a more powerful punch of nutrients than the old alternatives.

The following grains are all gluten-free. Later, I will compare the nutritional properties of G-free grains and gluten-containing grains. By building your diet around these power grains, you will be substantially boosting your vitamin and mineral intake every single day of the week.

Amaranth: Like quinoa, amaranth is sometimes referred to as a "pseudo-grain," because while it looks like (and cooks like) a grain, it's actually a seed that's related to spinach, beets, and pigweed. Amaranth is high in fiber, iron, calcium, and lysine. If you are a neat freak, however, I would stick with premade options with this grain, as baking with amaranth—which resembles those teeny round "sprinkles"—can be messy.

Arrowroot: Used for thickening soups and gravies, arrowroot is a powdery flour that resembles cornstarch.

Artichoke: Dried artichokes can be ground and used as flour in baked goods.

Bean flour: Bean flours are produced from pulverized dried or ripe beans. They can be made from all sorts of different beans. A few nutrient-packed examples:

- Chickpea flour: Chickpea flour, also known as besan, gram (*not* to be confused with glutenous graham flour), or channa flour, is used to make dumplings and noodles. Chickpea flatbreads and pancakes are popular in India, France, and Italy.
- Garfava flour: Garfava flour is a blend of chickpea flour and fava bean flour.
- Lentil flour: Lentil flour can also be used to make pancakes and other flatbreads.
- Soy flour: Another by-product of the versatile soybean, soy flour is a low-carb, high-protein alternative to traditional wheat flours.

Buckwheat: Despite its name (which I must admit still puts me off!), buckwheat has no relation to wheat, which makes it a safe

alternative for anyone avoiding the gluten grains. In fact, like quinoa, buckwheat isn't even a grain—it's a seed related to rhubarb and
sorrel. The health benefits of buckwheat are truly staggering: It's a
rich source of fiber, magnesium, all eight essential amino acids, and
even protein. Buckwheat also contains an antioxidant called rutin, a
flavonoid that can lower the risk of developing high cholesterol and
high blood pressure, as well as chiro-inositol, which drives carbohydrates into your muscles without raising insulin levels. As always,
just check that it hasn't been grown and processed near wheat.

Cassava: *See* Tapioca.

Corn: Flour made from corn (also known as maize, maiz, masa
harina) is a common cooking ingredient in the Southwestern
United States and in Mexico. Corn tortillas, polenta, and corn and
hominy grits all make great gluten substitutes.

- Cornmeal: Cornmeal is made from coarse whole-grain corn.
  Italian polenta is a cornmeal dish.
- Corn flour: Corn flour—which you can find in white, yellow,
  and blue varieties—is used to make cornbread, corn tortillas,
  and corn cereal.
- Cornstarch, modified cornstarch: Cornstarch is a versatile
  gluten-free thickener.

Flax meal, flax flour: Flax meal and flax flour, which are made from
ground-up flaxseeds, tend to be coarse and fibrous. While they're
pretty hard to cook with (as they can go rancid at high temperatures),
flax meal and flour are great for sprinkling over all sorts of other
foods: cereal, yogurt, smoothies, salads, puddings. Anytime you want
to enhance the nutritional value (and taste) of a food, reach for the
flaxseed. I will even add a few pinches of flax meal to pancake batter.

Manioc: *See* Tapioca.

Millet: Millet, which is not a grain but a grass, is nutrient-rich and easy to cook (and digest!). Just make sure it has *not* been processed near wheat.

Nut flours: Ground-up nuts of every description—almonds, hazelnuts, chestnuts, walnuts, peanuts—are the basis for a delicious variety of nut flours, which are often used in desserts. Nuts processed into oils and butters are also gluten-free.

Potato flour, potato starch flour: Potato flour and potato starch flour are often used to thicken foods.

Quinoa: The so-called "mother grain" in ancient Incan civilizations, quinoa is a tiny, beadlike seed that's a powerful source of protein and other essential nutrients. Like millet, quinoa is easy to cook and has a rich, nutty flavor.

Rice: Rice, a member of the grass family, is the most common cereal grain on the planet, ahead of even wheat. In its pure form, rice is always gluten-free. "Aromatic rice" is also G-free, but watch out for preflavored rice mixes and the sticky rice in sushi, both of which might contain added gluten. All of the following rice varieties are safe to eat:

- Arborio rice: Short-grained Arborio rice is the main ingredient in Italian risottos.
- Basmati rice: This long-grain rice is packed with flavor.
- Brown rice flour: Brown rice flour is a staple of Southeast Asian cooking. It is higher in nutrients than traditional white rice flour.
- Brown rice: Brown rice is less refined and more nutritious than white rice.
- Enriched rice: Enriched rice is white rice that has had some of the nutrients, mainly iron and the B vitamins, such as niacin and folic acid, restored after the milling process.

- Glutinous rice: A misnomer, according to Dr. Green. Despite the name, glutinous rice is G-free. Made by grinding short-grain rice, glutinous rice is used all over Asia to thicken sauces and add sweetness to desserts.
- Instant rice: Instant rice is G-free as long as it's unflavored. Quick-cooking rice that you boil in a bag contains no gluten unless the label indicates otherwise.
- Japonica rice.
- Jasmine rice: Aromatic jasmine rice is popular in Asia.
- Long-grain rice.
- Pearl rice.
- Polished rice.
- Popcorn rice.
- Rice bran.
- Rice couscous: Don't be led astray by the name. Rice couscous was named for its physical resemblance to gluten-containing couscous. But it's still rice, and contains no gluten.
- Risotto: *See* Arborio rice.
- Texmati: Texmati rice is another type of aromatic rice.
- White rice flour.
- Wild rice.

Tapioca: Tapioca is produced from the root of the cassava plant (which is also known as manioc, cassava, and yucca) and used to make sweet tapioca pudding. Tapioca can be used as a thickening agent in other foods as well. When blended with other G-free flours, it can make batter fluffier.

- Modified tapioca starch.
- Tapioca flour.

Sorghum: Sorghum, a G-free substitute for wheat flour, has been popular in Africa and India for centuries, and has recently attracted notice in this country as well. Sorghum can be made into a syrup, or fermented into alcoholic beverages.

Teff: Teff is the smallest grain in the world, and one of the most nutritious, too. It is the main ingredient in *injera*, the traditional Ethiopian flatbread.

Yucca: *See* Tapioca.

Other Basic Gluten-Free Food Groups

BREAKFAST FOODS

You can make all sorts of healthy hot breakfast cereals without gluten: for example, corn grits, hominy grits, and cream of rice. You can also have cereals made from puffed rice. Ashley Koff, RD, author of *Recipes for IBS*, suggests making a QuinteSensual bowl of quinoa. In "Resources," I have listed gluten-free commercial cereals, including ones for kids. My new favorite cereal is Perky's Nutty Flax—it seems like every time I hit the grocery store, I fall in love with a new treat!

Ashley Koff also has a number of alternatives to traditional pancakes in *Recipes for IBS*, which has recipes for sweet potato pancakes, lentil-amaranth pancakes, and sweet zucchini pancakes. You could also make G-free banana-nut pancakes by adding the nuts and banana to a gluten-free mix, or Rustic French Toast using G-free rice or millet breads.

MEAL-REPLACEMENT BARS

While it is far better to eat real food, this is not always an option in our busy world. You should stock up on various grab-and-go meal-replacement bars and shakes. In my search for the perfect bar, I have been working diligently. Some standbys are Lärabars and Biomedics bars. I list many more options in "Resources."

CANNED FOODS

Most canned foods are G-free if they contain only a single food (for example, beans or tomatoes). But as always, examine the label

Don't become *too* dependent on these and other ready-made foods. When I first got off gluten and was completely food-phobic, I fell into the habit of eating up to three protein bars every day: They were G-free, they tasted good, and they filled me up—what could be better? "It's perfectly normal to get into a rut with foods like this early on," Ashley Koff, RD, said. "Feeling comfortable with, and in control of, your food choices is a really important first step. But for the next phase, I would really recommend making the transition to as many whole foods as possible versus those in a bag or a box; this is a recommendation for optimal health to heal the digestive system (from years of gluten consumption) as well as reduce risk of chronic disease…Many processed foods contain preservatives that are unfamiliar to the body and, in their own way, harsh on the system.

"Many meal-replacement bars contain preservatives and modified ingredients such as sugar alcohols. Sugar alcohols, which are designed to offer a low-carb sugar profile, can present a challenge to the digestive system as they are not meant to be absorbed and as such often cause gas and irritation. So instead of helping the healing process, these sugar alcohols and other preservatives may further irritate," says Ashley Koff, RD.

She recommends eating soybeans in the whole food form (edamame, tofu, etc.) versus bars and other food products made with isolated soy protein. There are great nutrients in the whole bean, fiber, and omega-3 fatty acids, among others that are lost when we isolate the protein. Additionally, countries whose populations consume soy (and whose populations seem to reap the health benefits) are consuming the soy in a food form. There is some question about the role of soy protein isolate as helpful or harmful in cancer and other diseases. So grab an apple with almond butter, some edamame, or a mixture of nuts and seeds for a quick on-the-go snack—they are convenient, and your body will recognize and use every part of them efficiently and effectively.

until you are positive that no emulsifiers, preservatives, stabilizers, or undefined food starches have been added.

CHEESE

While all blue cheese (which gets its name from the moldy blue flecks that originated on bread) could contain gluten, most other hard cheeses like Parmesan and cheddar are gluten-free in their natural state. But like so many foods, cheese might come into contact with gluten at different points in the manufacturing and packaging process. Cheeses sliced and wrapped in the store could be contaminated with gluten, so I only buy cheeses that are prepackaged and clearly labeled gluten-free. (Kraft, among other companies, always labels its G-free cheeses.) Unless someone can confirm to me that a cheese is gluten-free, I stay away. I feel a lot safer with products that are explicitly labeled gluten-free.

COLD CUTS

You have several choices when it comes to buying cold cuts. You can buy prepackaged meats like Hormel Natural Choice, which are labeled gluten-free. Or you can get the person at your deli to slice your sandwich meat while you are standing there. If you go this route, you have to make sure that the meat slicer is completely wiped down and free of any traces of gluten. I recommend getting to the deli counter bright and early in the morning, when the lines are short and the slicer recently cleaned. It also helps to develop a personal relationship with the person behind your meat counter, so I suggest shopping at the same days and times if your schedule allows it. Leave yourself enough time to watch the slicer being cleaned. If you are in a hurry, you should probably just go for the prepackaged meats.

CONDIMENTS AND SALAD DRESSINGS

Many everyday condiments—Dijon mustard, Heinz ketchup—are gluten-free. You can also find a wide range of G-free salad dressings from companies such as Annie's Natural and Newman's Own. But do know that the single word "vinegar" on a salad dressing label can refer to a mixture of vinegars, some of which might contain gluten. In most cases, unless you see the words "gluten-free" on the label, you are going to have to call the company to find out the source of the vinegar. Low-fat salad dressings can also be risky, so verify all ingredients before tasting. You can always just whip up your own salad dressing from olive oil, balsamic vinegar, mustard, and lemon juice.

PIZZA CRUSTS AND TORTILLAS

For pizza crusts, you have options! In *Recipes for IBS*, Ashley Koff, RD, uses brown rice (you can also add chia seeds or flaxseeds) and polenta as pizza crust options. You can also purchase the G-free pizza crust mixes. To compensate for a different flavor or decrease in flavor (as perceived by some), try adding Parmesan cheese or spices to the dough mix, or spread oil and herbs/spices onto the dough along with the other toppings. You also have several alternatives to flour tortillas. You can make your own tortillas out of buckwheat flour (there is a great recipe for "Buck-the-Wheat" tortillas in *Recipes for IBS*), or you can use a corn tortilla.

SOUP BASES

Soon after I went G-free, I started making huge vats of Tim's mom's white chicken chili recipe to get us through the week. The chili tasted great, and I wasn't adding any gluten—so why did I always feel so sick after eating it? It took me several months to identify the culprit: The commercial soup stock I'd been using was filled with hidden glutens. So even though I *thought* I was making a G-free meal, I was inadvertently poisoning my body every time I dug into that chili. Avoid this common mistake, and choose your bouillon cubes and liquid soup stocks carefully; make sure they don't have any added glutens. There are plenty of safe choices out there. Pacific Foods and Health Valley both make gluten-free broths, and Herb-Ox and Edwards and Sons bouillon cubes are both gluten-free.

COFFEE AND TEA

Here I go again: Coffee and tea are gluten-free, but only in their *pure form*. Watch out in particular for flavored, instant, and decaffeinated coffees, all of which might contain gluten. You don't even want to have any coffee from a coffeemaker used for flavored coffees, as the residue can transfer from one pot to another. Wash out that coffeemaker several times before making your own beverage in it. I also wouldn't recommend drinking any coffee at weddings or other public events, since it's usually instant. Hotels also serve a lot of instant coffee. If you absolutely can't live without flavored coffee, Starbucks, Peet's, Ghirardelli, Folgers, and Dunkin' Donuts all brew up G-free coffees in every flavor under the sun—just call customer service to double-check.

BREADS, PASTAS, AND MIXES

Traditional breads and pastas are off-limits, but that's okay! There are *tons* of deliciously, nutritiously superior alternatives out there, with a wider selection available every day. In the "Resources," there are pages and pages of information on where to find delicious, G-free breads, from companies such as Valpiform Breads, Ener-G Foods, Glutino, Food for Life—and the list keeps growing. You can also buy ready-made bread mixes from Bob's Red Mill at most health food stores. Tinkyada makes a great brown rice pasta, and health food stores will usually stock a range of clear rice noodles, which are a staple of Asian cuisine. For a complete buying guide, refer to "Resources."

CHIPS AND OTHER SNACKS

You don't have to drive an hour to a specialty food store to get your hands on good chips and other essential snacking material. Do be careful, though, because some products that don't themselves contain gluten might pass on the same conveyor belt as wheat-containing foods—yet another reason you need to get into the habit of calling food manufacturers on a regular basis. After that unpleasant experience with my once-favorite brand of corn chips, I generally eat only chips that are labeled gluten-free, because those words generally indicate that more precautions have been taken to prevent cross-contamination. I like to snack without wondering how I am going to feel in an hour. I also love Pirate's Booty cheese puffs and Mary's Gone Crackers seed-and-rice crackers.

COOKIES, CANDIES, AND OTHER DESSERTS

The good news (and the bad news!) is that it's extremely easy to get your G-free sugar fix. A few suggestions:

Cookies: Pamela's Products cookies are a big hit at our house—one of the G-free treats that are quickest to vanish!

Candies: Lots of candies are G-free, even if they aren't labeled as such. Kit-Kat, Twix Bars, and other candy bars with a "cookie" component do contain gluten. The Foundation for Celiac Awareness (www.celiaccentral.org) updates their extensive list of G-free candies every October—just in time for Halloween! The most recent roundup includes 3 Musketeers, Baby Ruth, Bit-O-Honey, Butterfinger, Jelly Bellies (except buttered popcorn flavor), Hershey's

---

Healthier Alternative to Cookies

Purchasing an already-made gluten-free cookie raises the same issue as purchasing a regular already-made cookie. It's more likely to have preservatives and be more processed. Instead of a store-bought cookie, bake your own. Choose a gluten-free cookie mix, then you get to dress them up to you or your kids' taste preferences. Add nuts, spices, crystallized ginger, nut butter, fruit, coconut, or chocolate to make a delicious, more nutrient dense, and oh yes, gluten-free cookie or cookie bar. Freeze the dough or make some for the office. When choosing a ready-to-go cookie, use the same overall nutrition health guidelines (no partially hydrogenated oils, no high-fructose corn syrup, etc.) used to distinguish a better-quality product. Try the cashew-teff cookies in Ashley Koff's *Recipes for IBS*.

Kisses, Kraft Caramels, Mounds, Oh Henry, PayDay, Raisinets, Reese's Peanut Butter Cups, Rolo, Sour Patch Kids, Starburst Fruit Chews, Sugar Babies, Swedish Fish, Sweet Tarts, Tic Tacs, York Peppermint Patties…The list goes on and on! Not too shabby, right? But always check before buying a candy.

The candies that *do* contain gluten might surprise you. While pure licorice is G-free, lots of commercial licorice candies are not. Before learning about this distinction, I would eat strawberry licorice twists every time I went to the movies…and I would be racked by pain long before the closing credits scrolled down the screen. For years, I thought I was allergic either to the movies, or to my date!

Gelatin desserts and puddings: Kozy Shack rice and chocolate puddings (my favorite!) are G-free. Some pudding mixes, such as Jell-O, are as well—check with the manufacturer for confirmation.

Gum: Bubblicious Gum, Bubble Yum Gum, and all Wrigley's gum are gluten-free.

Healthier Alternative to Candy

Ashley Koff, RD, recommends that you make your own trail mix. Add different chips (peanut, chocolate), coconut, dried fruit—this offers many more nutrients than candy, which is low in nutrients and high in sugar and often high in fat as well.

Ice creams and sorbets: Since dairy products are naturally gluten-free, many ice creams are as well. Ben & Jerry's, Baskin-Robbins, and Edy's all have gluten-free options. Always avoid ice creams with wheat-based add-ins like cookies (or cookie dough), brownies, or pretzels. Ordering ice cream at a stand or in a store can be more complicated—see page 131 for a rundown of how to handle those situations.

FROZEN MEALS

Keep your freezer filled with ready-to-eat foods that you can pop into the microwave and enjoy at a moment's notice, when your family is ordering in, or when you are visiting someone whom you know well enough to use her microwave! Stock up on frozen soups, frozen pizzas, frozen desserts, frozen breads—anything you might need to get you through a pinch. Enjoy Life Foods and Amy's Kitchen both make terrific G-free ready meals.

Before you know it, you will find that there are many more foods that you *can* eat than ones you cannot!

Action Checklist
- To find out if a food contains gluten, do most of your legwork *before* going to the store.
- Research product ingredients on the Internet, and by calling the manufacturer directly.

If You Like...	Then Try:
Pad Thai noodles	Rice noodles or spaghetti squash
Quesadillas	Greensadilla (from *Recipes for IBS*), or a G-free tortilla
Breaded fish	G-free crab cakes (from *Recipes for IBS*)
Wrap or roll-up sandwiches	Rice paper wrappers (Crab-Pomegranate rolls for pizza roll-ups from *Recipes for IBS*)
Wheat crackers	Veggie chips from zucchinis, radishes, and sweet potatoes, or Xochitl corn chips. You can also use mini red potatoes (from *Recipes for IBS*)
Sweet dessert bars	Halvah (from *Recipes for IBS* or store-bought), berry rice pudding, or Pamela's chocolate-chip cookies

Courtesy of Ashley Koff, RD.

- Review the synonyms for gluten in Chapter 4 to familiarize yourself with terms you might see on a label.
- Familiarize yourself with all the naturally G-free foods out there, and be creative in seeking out healthier G-free alternatives to your once-favorite foods.
- Experiment with the range of G-free flours out there.

8

G-Free Home Cooking

Now that you know how to shop, you are ready for the next big step on the road to G-*free*dom: learning to prepare your own food. The kitchen is your next frontier, the place where you can explore countless foods that you never even knew existed. Worry not: Learning to cook without gluten does not mean reinventing the wheel. As long as you are willing to experiment with different styles of cooking, you can look forward to some incredible culinary adventures.

Technical Tips

TIP 1: MASTER A FEW EASY DISHES

Even if you are not a five-star chef, you should learn how to prepare a few simple, nourishing meals at a moment's notice. After all, only in your own kitchen can you be 100 percent positive that the food you are eating is safe and free from contamination. So while it's always good to have a few frozen dinners on hand, you also need to eat a variety of fresh foods.

Whether it's beans and rice, a chicken breast with steamed veggies, or a quinoa stew, you should work on mastering some easy-to-make recipes that you can throw together on a busy weeknight. You could also make some favorite dishes on a Sunday night and freeze what you don't eat for the week. (I wish I had the discipline to do this for myself!)

If you are interested in expanding your repertoire, I recommend investing in a few cookbooks that focus on gluten-free cooking, like *Beyond Rice Cakes* by Vanessa Maltin or *The Best Gluten-Free Family Cookbook* by Donna Washburn and Heather Butt. Ashley Koff's *Recipes for IBS* has some great menu ideas as well. You might also consider picking up some international cookbooks, since many countries cook with much less gluten than we do. Learning to make a simple Chinese stir-fry or a corn enchilada casserole could be a big timesaver. Before long, it may also become a family favorite!

TIP 2: LET YOUR CREATIVITY RUN WILD (AND DON'T WORRY ABOUT OCCASIONAL DUDS!)

Throw out everything you thought you knew about cooking and especially baking—it's a whole new world out there. Get acquainted with G-free grains such as millet and cornmeal, and improvise with updates of old favorite dishes. Does your favorite marinara sauce taste the same on rice pasta as it did on wheat? Does it need more basil, or another drop of olive oil? Trial and error is your new best friend, so don't be afraid of failure, especially in the beginning. The best chefs in the world have all had their share of culinary mishaps. And who knows—you might even enjoy cooking *more* than you did before. It really can be entertaining to investigate which ingredients will stick together without the help of that universal binder, gluten…You will soon be amazed.

TIP 3: IS IT DONE YET?

When you are cooking or baking G-free, cultivate the art of patience. This can be really hard, especially since you have waited so long to find ingredients that will not hurt you. That G-free cake will seem like it is taking *forever* to cook. And it is certainly true that gluten-free foods often take a little longer to cook than their glutenous counterparts. G-free flours tend to be much denser and slower to rise, so you should consider using smaller circular pans. Most gluten-free cookbooks have general guidelines to follow, and as you experiment, you will start to discover for yourself what works and what does not. Believe me: It is always worth the wait.

TIP 4: FALL IN LOVE WITH G-FREE FLOURS AND MIXES!

When I was little, I'd sit and watch my great-grandmother make her famous Italian biscuits. I'd help her twist the dough, or paint the tops with egg or oil. The aroma of the biscuits fresh out of the oven would rise up from the basement, where she made them, to my room on the third floor of the apartment. Those after-noons are still as fresh in my mind as the ingredients were in my great-grandmother's hands.

Though I was not a frequent baker even at the height of my gluten-eating days, after my diagnosis I wondered if I'd ever be able to pass these wonderful traditions on to my own children. Ever since my daughter, Grace, could hold a spoon, she has loved to bake. There is nothing more precious than the moments we have shared in the kitchen, baking a cake together. By the same token, there is nothing more *heartbreaking* than mixing a cake batter with your daughter and then waving her off when she sticks a spatula in your face and asks you to taste it. Let me tell you: It's almost impossible for me to reject a little cutie covered in frosting, even if I know that "taste" will come back to haunt me. To avoid these situations—and also to expand the range of foods I can make for myself—I've become more of a gluten-free baker because sharing in the moment, with kids, often means literally sharing in the moment.

There are a number of alternatives to gluten-containing flours and fillers out there. You can experiment with various combinations of amaranth and arrowroot, sorghum and soy. Many G-free cookbooks go into detail about substituting G-free flours in your favorite recipes. In keeping with your new improvisational spirit, start mixing and matching flours as the mood strikes, and have fun figuring out which combinations you and your family like best. There may even come a time when something will taste so good that no one will even know it is G-free!

You can also just take advantage of all the premixed gluten-free flours now on the market. When I first went off gluten, there were virtually no ready-made flours and cake mixes in supermarkets, so I still get a kick out of buying mixes that I can whip into a cake in a matter of minutes. Arrowhead Mills makes an all-purpose baking mix, a blend of organic whole-grain brown rice flour, potato starch, tapioca starch flour, and fava bean flour that you can use to whip up just about anything. They also make a G-free brownie mix, pancake and waffle mix, cookie mix, pizza crust mix—the possibilities are endless.

Kathy Burger loves the Baking and Pancake Mix made by Pamela's Products. "Whenever I hear someone has a gluten allergy," she said, "I tell them to buy that mix, and buy it in bulk. We make [our four-year-old daughter] Katie pancakes with that, we make her waffles with that, we make muffins with that. The chocolate-chunk cookie recipe on the baking mix box is the best one. The best one by far—they taste like regular chocolate chip cookies."

Kathy also likes the Whole Foods brand gluten-free baking mix. "I searched and I searched," she said, "and it's the one that tastes the most like normal cake. When I serve it at a party, nobody even notices that it's gluten-free. We make it with Stonyfield Yogurt, and it's *really* good." For parties outside the home, Kathy bakes

---

Reminder: Cross-Contamination

As always when cooking G-free, you need to make sure that all surfaces and cooking tools are clean and free of any gluten residue. You can never be too careful, even in your own kitchen!

---

large quantities of both vanilla and chocolate cupcakes. "I make a big batch of chocolate and a big batch of vanilla," she said, "and then I wrap each one individually and put them in a bag in the freezer." Whenever Katie is leaving for a party, Kathy calls ahead and finds out what is being served so that her daughter can enjoy a similar-looking treat.

Cooking for Your Family

Eating is one of the most social, intimate activities there is, an experience to be shared and savored with the people you love most in the world every single day of the week. Hanging out in the kitchen, trading bites of dessert, sampling new recipes, swiping food off the cutting board before it's ready to be served—these are all irreplaceable parts of family life.

So, should your family members give up gluten when you do? That's not a question anyone else can answer for you. I wonder what we would do if one of our kids was diagnosed with celiac disease, if we would clear our kitchen of every last breadcrumb that same day. So far, I am happy to say that day hasn't come. And for now, since there are three of them and only one of me, I have no desire to deprive my favorite people of their favorite foods—that's why we have a "compromised kitchen."

Of course, every household is different, and every decision hinges on a range of factors. But no matter how you choose to proceed, you should always feel totally comfortable in your own kitchen. Make your family members your allies on your gluten-free journey.

TIP 1: ROME WASN'T BUILT IN A DAY!

A celiac disease diagnosis can come as a major shock—especially to your family members. Your condition will dramatically change *all* of your lives no matter what, so you have a lot to gain by making your family's transition as smooth as possible. Though you may have to overhaul *your* diet overnight, your family members might need a little more time to adjust. Give them that time, opting for gradual modifications over harsh, all-or-nothing measures. Teach them about your new diet, and as you learn new tricks of the trade, include them in both your triumphs and your flops. Just don't expect instant compliance with your G-free lifestyle. In the years to come, your loved ones will make constant sacrifices on your behalf, deferring to your comfort level when it comes to choosing everything from restaurants to birthday cakes. It's important to acknowledge that the changes can be just as intimidating for them as they are for you. You will all figure it out together.

TIP 2: REINVENT FAMILY FAVORITES—MINUS THE GLUTEN

Devising gluten-free versions of your old standby meals is a wonderful way to satisfy your family members *and* your small intestine. My mom makes a lasagna that tastes *exactly* like the one I had growing up—the first time I tried it, I just couldn't believe gluten-free pasta could taste that good. Nor could I thank my mom enough for making such an effort on my behalf. With a little research and a lot of TLC, you can find ways of adapting your old recipes into meals that your whole family can enjoy together.

You could also try what my husband calls the "throw the dog a bone" approach. Rather than making the rest of your family a meal that's off-limits to you, try cooking a G-free meal for everyone, then adding a roll or a side dish of pasta. That way, you get to eat exactly what your family members are eating without depriving them of their beloved flaky biscuits.

TIP 3: SERVE FIRST; EXPLAIN LATER

As your G-free cooking skills improve, you might find that it gets easier and easier to feed your family gluten-free meals—without a single cringe. Often, people are more open-minded about new foods *after* they've tasted them. So surprise your family members—and don't hesitate to be sneaky! The other night, when Tim was raving about these fishsticks I'd served, I couldn't stop smiling: He had absolutely no idea they were gluten-free until the meal was over. Would he have been as enthusiastic if I'd revealed my secret before he took his first bite? I think not!

TIP 4: TRY NOT TO FALL INTO THE TRAP OF THE MADE-TO-ORDER MOMMY

Too often, I find myself, like many, slipping into the role of what I call "restaurant mommy," meaning I am making every member of my family an entirely different dinner. I will make Tim my special jalapeño-chili mac-and-cheese, then a kid version (i.e., minus the jalapeño, plus a little chicken) for Grace. By the time I am done feeding Taylor, I am lucky if I have the energy to pop a frozen dinner in the microwave for myself.

No working parent can handle this juggling act for long. So whenever possible, simplify your life by making everyone's meal gluten-free. My favorite nights, I make everyone happy with gluten-free pasta, fajitas, or tacos with corn tortillas. (This last dish is one of our family favorites, since we all prefer dishes that don't *scream* G-free at you.) So keep experimenting with various G-free crowd-pleasers. Over time, your family members will develop their own G-free favorites, and your job will be a good deal less exhausting.

Cooking for Crowds

You can adopt several different tactics when having people over for dinner.

Option 1: Make a G-free dinner for everyone. (And just as I take pleasure in occasionally fooling my family members, I love serving dinner guests an entirely G-free meal without mentioning what it does—or rather does *not*—contain. I see how long I can go before letting people in on my secret ingredients!) The more you experiment with gluten-free cooking, the better you will get at whipping up show-stopping meals not just for your family, but for dinner guests as well. If you have the time, I'd really recommend using dinner parties as an excuse to show off your brilliant G-free cooking skills.

Option 2: You might decide to make a *mostly* gluten-free meal and serve it with a side dish of pasta or bread—the "throw the dog a bone" approach. If you go this modified route, always pay attention to the placement of glutenous foods in relation to your plate. Or if you are too busy to prepare an elaborate G-free meal ahead of time, you can steal one of my favorite entertaining tricks and put on what I call the "indoor barbecue." I will just serve corn on the cob, watermelon, grilled chicken (in a G-free marinade, of course!), and salad. Your guests can help themselves to buns—just keep them out of contact with your food, by taking your pieces first and *then* setting them out for everyone else.

Option 3: If you are superrushed, make your guests a quick G-full meal and then microwave your own snack right before you sit down to the table. This isn't ideal, but sometimes it is just plain easier. As always when serving mixed meals, keep your gluten-free foods separate, and avoid community bowls.

TIP 5: IF YOU *ARE* MAKING SEPARATE MEALS FOR DIFFERENT FAMILY MEMBERS, ALWAYS COOK THE G-FREE VERSION FIRST

This commonsense precaution will really simplify the task of cooking separate meals for yourself and the rest of your household, if that's what you choose to do. If you make the gluten-free meal first, on clean surfaces, then you don't have to clean up the kitchen before getting started on the gluten-containing meal. You can't boil wheat pasta in a pot and then use that same pot to make rice, but there's no reason why you can't make the G-full pasta in the same pot that you already used for the G-free version. By cooking the G-free meal first, you don't have to worry so much about separating your pots, pans, and cooking utensils.

TIP 6: SET THE TABLE STRATEGICALLY

Over time, strategically positioning your plate will become second nature to you. When setting the table, make sure that your plate is as far away as possible from the breadbasket. If the breadbasket is going to be passed around the table, make sure that it goes around your plate: You don't want to be in the middle of that flight pattern. And if you are setting out food for company, make sure that there's no gluten between the G-free chips and salsa. Crumbs travel.

Family Recipes

My mom sent me her special G-free adaptations of our family's favorite Italian recipes.

Meat-Based Tomato Sauce for Baked Penne and Lasagna

This is my mother's basic meat sauce, which I use and which she and my grandmother used, over penne, spaghetti, and other pasta. My mother adapted it and the meatballs to make them gluten-free for me. I serve the meatballs and sausage on the side, with a fresh garden salad. I use this meat sauce for the baked penne recipe that follows, and also for lasagna.

The recipe calls for sausage, but a piece of pork, such as a thick boneless pork chop, can be substituted. Pork gives tomato sauce nice dimension. I make the meatballs small so that the sauce penetrates them during simmering, keeping them moist.

Time savers: *I sometimes make the meatballs ahead, and refrigerate or freeze them until I am ready to make the sauce. Sometimes I make the sauce ahead, and refrigerate or freeze it until I am ready to make the baked penne.*

1 pound Italian sausage, gluten-free, hot or sweet
1 small onion
3 tablespoons light olive oil or canola oil
3 28-ounce cans crushed tomatoes
1 teaspoon sugar
1 teaspoon salt
1/2 teaspoon fresh ground black pepper
3 or 4 fresh basil leaves
meatballs, gluten-free, cooked (recipe follows)

Cut the sausage into 2-inch pieces, and set aside. Mince the onion in a food processor, and set aside.

Heat the oil in a Dutch oven or large pot, and brown the sausage on all sides in the oil. Add the onion and cook it with the sausage until the onion is soft and light brown.

Add 1 can of crushed tomatoes to the pot. Add about 1/4 can of water to rinse the can and add the water to the pot. Stir, scraping the brown bits from the bottom of the pan. Add the other 2 cans of tomatoes, rinsing each can with 1/4 can of water and adding the water to the pot. Add the sugar, salt, pepper, and basil, and stir to mix. Add the meatballs and stir.

Bring the sauce to a boil over medium-high heat, stirring occasionally; then lower the heat to a slow simmer. Simmer sauce for 30 minutes or longer if desired. I like to simmer the sauce until I see that oil has risen to the top. Stir occasionally to prevent sticking.

Serve over pasta, or use in baked penne, or in lasagna. Note: I often use a Crock-Pot to make this sauce. If you use a Crock-Pot, brown the sausage and onion in a large skillet. Add the cooked sausage and onion to the Crock-Pot, using water to scrape up the brown bits with them. Add the remaining ingredients according to the above directions, and stir. Cook on HI for 4–5 hours, then switch to LO for 1–2 hours or until ready to use. Or cook on LO for 7–8 hours.

Meatballs

1/2 cup hominy grits or coarse cornmeal (or 1/2 cup gluten-free breadcrumbs)
1 1/2 pounds ground chuck
1 egg
1 garlic clove, minced
2 tablespoons chopped fresh parsley
2 tablespoons grated Romano or Parmesan cheese
1 teaspoon salt
1/4 teaspoon pepper

In a small bowl, combine 1 1/2 tablespoons of water to grits or cornmeal (or gluten-free breadcrumbs). Mix to moisten the grits or cornmeal (or gluten-free breadcrumbs), which should be damp, but not wet. Set aside. If using gluten-free rice crumbs, which are harder than cornmeal, use 1/4 cup of water and allow rice crumbs to soften for several minutes.

Place ground chuck in a large bowl. Add the egg, garlic, parsley, grated cheese, salt, and pepper, and mix with a wooden spoon. Add the moistened grits or cornmeal (or gluten-free breadcrumbs) and mix, first with the spoon, and then with your hands, just until ingredients are combined.

Shape the meat mixture into meatballs, about the size of golf balls.

Brown the meatballs in a skillet in light olive oil or canola oil. Cook in batches, and do not overcrowd the skillet. Add more oil if needed. Remove the meatballs from the skillet and set aside for use in the tomato sauce, or cover and refrigerate or freeze until you are ready to make the tomato sauce.

Baked Penne with Meat Sauce

1 pound gluten-free penne or ziti
12–16-ounce ball of low-moisture mozzarella cut into
　　1/2-inch cubes, or 12–16 ounces shredded mozzarella
3/4 cup grated Romano or Parmesan cheese
meatballs and sausage from the tomato sauce
3–4 cups tomato sauce (recipe above)

Preheat oven to 375 degrees.

Remove half of the meatballs and half of the sausage pieces from the tomato sauce. Slice the meatballs and the sausage, and set aside.

Add 1 teaspoon of salt to a large pot of water, and bring to a boil. Add the penne or ziti and cook for about 6 or 7 minutes. The pasta should be harder than al dente because the pasta will continue to cook when baked. Strain the pasta, and return it to the pot.

Add about 2 cups of tomato sauce to the pasta, and mix with a wooden spoon until the sauce is evenly distributed. Add the mozzarella cheese and the grated cheese to the pasta, reserving 2 tablespoons of each for topping. Mix with the spoon. Add the slices of meatballs and sausage, reserving 1/3 cup of each for topping. Mix gently with the wooden spoon.

Spoon about 1/2 cup of tomato sauce onto the bottom of a lasagna pan or a 9×13-inch baking dish. Spoon the pasta and meat mixture into the pan or baking dish. Spread the reserved slices of meatballs and sausage over the pasta. Spoon a thin layer of sauce over the top of the pasta and meat toppings. Be sure the sauce reaches the corners. Sprinkle the reserved mozzarella, and then the reserved grated cheese over the sauce. Cover with aluminum foil.

Bake the penne or ziti until the corners bubble, about 30–40 minutes. Remove the foil and bake uncovered for 7–10 minutes.

Remove the baked penne or ziti from the oven, cover with foil, and let it stand for 10 minutes before cutting and serving. Cut into squares (like lasagna) and serve with extra grated cheese and warm tomato sauce on the side, if desired.

Buon apetito!

Lasagna

1 pound container ricotta cheese
1 egg
1/4 cup chopped fresh parsley
1/2 cup hominy grits or coarse cornmeal (or 1/2 cup
   gluten-free breadcrumbs)
1 1/2 teaspoons salt
1/2 teaspoon fresh ground black pepper
pinch of cinnamon, optional
meatballs and sausage from the tomato sauce
12–16-ounce ball of low-moisture mozzarella cut into
   1/2-inch cubes, or 12–16 ounces shredded mozzarella

3/4 cup grated Romano or Parmesan cheese
1 tablespoon olive oil or canola oil
1 1/2 pounds gluten-free lasagna noodles
3–4 cups tomato sauce (see pages 104–5 for recipe)

Preheat oven to 375 degrees.

In a large bowl, mix together ricotta cheese, egg, parsley, grits or coarse cornmeal (or gluten-free breadcrumbs), 1/2 teaspoon salt, pepper, and cinnamon (if using). Set aside. If using gluten-free rice crumbs, which are harder than cornmeal, add 1/4 cup of water and allow rice crumbs to soften for several minutes.

Remove half of the meatballs and half of the sausage pieces from the tomato sauce. Slice the meatballs and the sausage, and set aside.

Set aside and reserve (for topping the lasagna) 2 tablespoons of the mozzarella and 2 tablespoons of the grated cheese.

Add 1 teaspoon of salt and 1 tablespoon of olive oil or canola oil (to prevent the noodles from sticking) to a large pot of water, and bring to a boil. Add the lasagna noodles and cook for about 6–7 minutes. The noodles should be harder than al dente because the noodles will continue to cook when baked. Strain the noodles in a colander.

While the pasta is cooking, spoon about 1/2 cup of tomato sauce onto the bottom of a lasagna pan or a 9×13-inch baking dish.

Place a layer of cooked lasagna noodles over the sauce in the lasagna pan or baking dish. Drop spoonfuls of 1/3 of the ricotta mixture on the layer of noodles and spread the mixture. Add 1/3 of the meatballs and sausage over the ricotta. Spread 1/3 of the shredded or cubed mozzarella as the next layer. Next spread on top of the meat and cheese layers about 1/3 cup of the tomato sauce, and sprinkle 1/3 of the grated cheese on the sauce.

Make a second layer of cooked lasagna noodles, and add the ricotta, meatballs and sausage, cheeses, and tomato sauce as above.

Repeat the process to make a third layer of lasagna noodles and meat and cheese fillings.

Cover the last layer of fillings with a layer of cooked lasagna noodles. Spoon a thin layer of sauce over the top of the lasagna noodles. Be sure the sauce reaches the corners. Sprinkle the reserved mozzarella and then the reserved grated cheese over the sauce. Cover with aluminum foil.

Bake the lasagna until the corners bubble, about 30–40 minutes. Remove the foil and bake uncovered for 7–10 minutes.

Remove the baked lasagna from the oven, cover with foil, and let it stand for 10 minutes before cutting and serving. Cut into squares and serve with extra grated cheese and warm tomato sauce on the side, if desired.

Buon appetito!

Action Checklist

- Start with simple dishes first. You can move on to more elaborate fare after you feel more comfortable in the kitchen.
- Never fear failure! Be patient with yourself and just keep on experimenting with G-free cooking and baking. You will get there.
- Try to find G-free versions of old family favorites. It helps if you serve the food *before* revealing its contents.
- Throwing dinner parties should not be daunting—you have as many entertaining choices as ever, possibly even more!

How Not to Be a Party Pooper

Having people over to dinner presents one set of challenges. Having dinner at someone else's house is another game altogether. To begin with, I should say that, with so many variables involved, there are really no do-or-die rules that universally apply to every social situation. As every relationship, circumstance, and comfort level is unique, so is the remedy to an awkward situation.

I admit that I still experience a certain level of anxiety when I am on my way to a dinner party, wedding, or any other sort of public event involving food. It's hard not to feel constantly under attack as a million paranoid questions run through my mind: What if my hosts think I am rude for refusing their food? What if my diet is the topic of conversation all night long? How can I have fun without keeling over in pain afterward? Where is the closest bathroom if things go wrong?

Even if I decide to throw caution to the wind and dig in (and I definitely don't recommend this!), I end up obsessively worrying about how I am going to feel by the end of the night. Needless to say, it's not exactly the recipe for an enjoyable evening.

Luckily, the right information will get you through the evening intact. As in all other aspects of your life, you just have to work out certain strategies before heading off to any social event, large or small.

Whether you are dining in a posh new restaurant or in your new coworker's backyard, you *can* safely venture out of your home and, yes, even have a normal social life without getting glutened at every turn!

As I share with you the techniques that have served me well over the years, always bear in mind that your approach really will depend on where you are, and in whose company you will be. As you learn to navigate the G-free universe on your own, you will develop your own tricks to ensure that your nights out are both fun *and* easy on the stomach. After all, the only thing worse than a party pooper is an *after*-party pooper.

Our goal: To be neither one!!!! These tips will help:

Tip 1: Pre-Party . . . At Home First

Some people save up all day for a big dinner party, skipping lunch so they can chow down that evening. You should take the exact opposite approach: Never, *ever* go to a dinner party or event hungry. Instead, I will eat immediately before leaving home, or on the way there. In general, it's safe to assume that when I enter your house, I am already happily full. If the food served happens to be G-free, excellent; if it's not, I hardly notice, since I am already stuffed. Eating in advance is a sure-fire way to stay out of trouble when you are out of your comfort zone.

Tip 2: BYOT! Bring Your Own (G-Free) Treat

Bringing your own little snack to any event lasting more than a couple of hours is always a good idea, but how you decide to go about doing this is entirely up to you. These two very different strategies have worked best for me over the years:

THE SOCIAL BUTTERFLY STRATEGY

Often, regardless of the situation, I find it easier on everyone to arrive at the party with a G-free snack and beverage in arms. I simply walk in the door, whip out my G-free chips and salsa, and say very casually, "Hey, I can't eat things that have gluten in them, so I brought my own treats for everyone to share." Because I've usually already pigged out before leaving home, a little snack is more than enough to get me through the most epic of dinner parties. I also recommend that you BYOB, like Redbridge gluten-free beer or Chopin potato vodka because it will have people trying something new, too! Most hosts certainly won't discourage your showing up with an extra snack.

THE SHRINKING VIOLET STRATEGY

On other occasions, you just will not be in the mood to explain your allergy and show up with a party pack. Or you might be leaving for an event straight from work, and you will not have the time to prepare a snack to bring along. Or you might just forget!

On these nights, your best bet is to stash a snack secretly in your bag or jacket that you can munch on secretly throughout the night! I will confess that I have many a time "stepped out" to eat a G-free snack (almonds, a protein bar, apple) in the car, bathroom, hallway, or any other secluded corner where I can nibble in peace!

THE BUDDY STRATEGY

This method works well at sit-down, banquet-style affairs, where meals are prepared in advance for large groups of people. I always "buddy up" with Tim. After stealing off for a G-free snack, I sit there, my plate untouched, until he has eaten about half of his meal. Then, when no one is looking, we swap plates lightning-fast! Tim happily starts his meal over, and I am off the hook.

The plate-swap trick does not always work, however. When Tim and I were heading to the White House for a state dinner with Queen Elizabeth, I told him that we would have to exercise *extreme* discretion when doing the plate swap. But then, once we got there, we were seated at different tables! I wasn't about to offend anybody, and I was already on such a high from sitting at the same table with the First Lady, Prince Charles, and Condoleezza Rice that I ate every bite of the food served me…and felt no pain afterward! My adrenaline completely eclipsed my tummy troubles on that once-in-a-lifetime evening.

Tip 3: Explain the Pain…But Do *Not* Let It Become the Topic of the Night!

Okay, so let's assume you've decided not to tell your hosts about your diet in advance. You've had a big bowl of G-free pasta before hitting the road, and you've successfully smuggled your own snack into the event. Now what? Again, you can adopt several different strategies depending on the type of event.

THE QUICK CHANGE OF SUBJECT

If you do get separated from your buddy and decide not to risk it, the people around you might ask why you are not eating. Or you might be busted with chocolate from your protein bar in the corner of your mouth…while everyone else is eating salad—what to do then? The key here: Be brief, be firm, and then briskly change the subject! For example, you can say, "I have a serious food allergy, so I just munch on this protein bar and I am good to go! Hey, did anyone see the Seahawks game last night? Amazing!" Whatever you do, do not let people dwell on your diet—it's just no way to enjoy your night out.

Rule of Thumb

Avoid community bowls. Take even *more* precautions when you are outside of your home. Stay far away from any bowl that might be contaminated with gluten. That means salsa, vegetable dips, queso, and so on are all off-limits.

FULL DISCLOSURE...IF YOU DARE!

Before accepting an invitation, you should weigh the pros and cons of prepping your host about your diet. As I've already mentioned, every situation is totally different, and only your own judgment can guide you.

But as people—especially parents of young children—are becoming more tuned in to the prevalence of food allergies, it's becoming increasingly common for hosts to ask about special dietary needs when issuing the invitation. If asked outright, I will definitely say that I can't eat gluten and go into some detail about what that means. But I will emphasize that the host is under *no* obligation to prepare a special meal for me.

I say this for my host, but also for *me*! Being honest is not always a guarantee of a relaxing, G-free evening—not by a long shot. Bringing up your diet can create two big issues. The first: Who wants to be a high-maintenance guest? Pulling off a successful social event is difficult enough without having to cater to one person's special needs, and the last thing you want is for your host to regret inviting you!

The second, more serious pitfall of mentioning your gluten allergy ahead of time is the possibility that your host will go out of her way to make you some extraspecial food that you *still* can't eat. There are so many hidden ingredients in foods, and so much the general public still does not know about cross-contamination. What if your host cooks up a special dish of G-free noodles but does not realize that

Most of my family and good friends know me well enough now to tell me what they are making, to ask me what snacks I would like, or to know that I may hesitate to take a bite of something when coming over for a party or dinner. But there have been many times, particularly when first getting to know someone, when I am thankful to have made my G-free status known.

- I always think back to when we first moved to Los Angeles and had met a great family at church. They asked us over one day for a bite. I mentioned, in the most casual way possible, that I have a gluten allergy, and when we got there, Kristy had made an entire plate of G-free pasta just for me! It blew me away to think that someone I had only briefly met would go so far out of her way to include me in the meal.

- In my first year or two on the show, my executive producer, Bill Geddie, and his wife, Barbara, asked me and Tim over for a home-cooked meal. Barbara had called ahead to see if there was anything I couldn't eat. "Do you have a pen?" I remember saying, only half in jest. After taking a moment to consider whether or not to trouble her, I spilled the beans. Because it would be the four of us at dinner, I knew that not eating any of what she had worked hard to make would be not only rude, but also incredibly obvious. I told her everything, then added that I'd bring a little something that I could eat, so she wouldn't have to worry. Upon arrival, she went through all of her ingredients with me over some great wine, and I felt at ease immediately.

- This past year, Whoopi Goldberg mentioned she was going to have a party for the entire "*View*" crew." She and her business partner, Tommy, asked about my allergy. I told them, but made sure to add that I in *no* way wanted anything special: "I come for the company," I said, "not for the food." When I arrived,

(*continued*)

everyone was raving about the impressive P.F. Chang's spread. Whoopi came over and walked me into the kitchen, where a separate tin of all G-free options was clearly labeled—just for me. It was one party where I hardly said a word, as my mouth was happily stuffed the entire night!

you can't use the same colander for the regular and the gluten-free pastas? What if the knife used to make my fruit salad was also used to slice the bread? What if I can't get out of bed tomorrow morning?

The sad truth is, even the best-intentioned host could inadvertently gluten you. That's why, in many instances, I feel more comfortable bringing my own foods to dinner parties, or just sneaking off into the bathroom to eat one of my G-free bars.

Tip 4: Ask Questions—If You Dare

All right, so your host knows all about your special diet and has gone out of her way to accommodate you—but does that necessarily mean that the food being served is safe? Do you interrogate her about her cooking methods, or simply roll the dice out of politeness? (I tend toward the latter approach.)

To the greatest extent possible, you should go out of your way to avoid these sticky situations. If presented with a questionable food, rely on your own best judgment. But if the host is a relative or a fairly close friend, don't be afraid to ask questions. Say, "Okay, great, so tell me how you did this! Walk me through the process." I will ask what they used to grease the pan: Cooking spray? Butter? Olive oil? (I am still suspicious of the "grain alcohol" listed in certain commercial cooking sprays, and if they used butter, what if the butter has been contaminated by gluten-containing breads?)

So what to do? Again, you have to make that decision for yourself:

Only you can know exactly what effect a food will have on you. For me, even if I am not 100 percent reassured that the food is safe, I will pretty much always taste anything that's been prepared especially for me. If someone makes me, say, G-free corn muffins, I *will* try one because I am just so grateful and moved by such an incredible act of thoughtfulness—and I barely have time to make those for myself anymore! So I just say a prayer and start chewing! Often, yes, I do suffer for this, but in some cases, this little leap of faith can be worth it.

One more thing: Note that this Q&A process *only* applies to foods that your host has assured you are G-free. If someone tries to foist plain old G-full pasta on you, or a batch of regular chocolate chip cookies, you are under *no* obligation to eat the food. On the contrary, you *are* under an obligation *not* to eat it.

Tip 5: Don't Take a Bite Just to Be Polite!

Okay, okay, I admit that I myself am guilty of doing this, but only when someone has made something G-free just for me. But what about when you are *certain* that a food contains gluten, or if your host pressures you? How many times have you heard people say, "Oh, one bite won't hurt you—just try it"? (Somehow, family members can be the most stubborn.) The only advice I can offer: Submit to peer pressure at your own peril. If given a food that you *know* will leave you clutching your abdomen for the next week, just say no! Even if your host keeps insisting that you try her famous pound cake (one taste couldn't possibly hurt!), hold your ground. Devoted friends will understand that you are declining not out of rudeness, but of medical necessity.

Tip 6: Just Say No—Politely!

Say someone offers you homemade cookies that you *know* will leave you reeling. How do you Just Say No without angering your host?

Survival Guide: The G-Free Wedding Guest

Think about the monumental effort that goes into planning a wedding. Brides and grooms to be have a million tiny details to manage without having to take a single guest's special needs into account.

In other words: You should *never* expect a person planning a wedding to order a separate gluten-free meal for you. It is *not* your day.

Besides, since when did anyone ever attend a wedding just for the food? You can still party with the best of 'em without partaking of the hors d'oeuvres platters. Focus instead on the great music, drinks, and reunion with old friends at the reception—there will be more than enough to distract you from that red velvet cake! I have, on a few occasions, been wonderfully surprised by a G-free meal prepared especially for me, like at a good friend's wedding. I am still thankful that even with their long to-do list, the bride and groom found time to think of me.

There are reasons beyond mere politeness to skip the meal portion of the big event. Even if the soon-to-be husband and wife make special allowances for you (And I repeat: Even if the bride is your best friend, do *not* specify that you have an allergy on the reply card!), you can never be totally confident that the food you are served will be safe. It is perfectly justifiable to remain a little apprehensive in any situation where food is being prepared in large quantities. (Never forget this at banquet dinners!) Even if the diligent waiter remembers to leave the bread roll off your plate, how can you know that your plain chicken breast has not crossed paths with dozens of other gluten-containing substances in preparation, or on the way to your table?

In the end, you should make all the same preparations for a wedding that you would for any other social situation:

Tip 1: Never leave the house hungry. In fact, I suggest leaving full. You will burn it all off on the dance floor! Eat as if you are about to go into hibernation, because by the time that last dance is done, if you are half-starving, the cranks will inevitably set in, and it will *not* be pretty.

Tip 2: Pack snacks. Fill your purse with almonds, candies, maybe a sandwich—whatever foods will keep you well fed and happy through-out the event. Low blood sugar moments and feeling starved will make for zero fun. To get through, I typically choose a clutch that can fit my go-to-G-free stash. When the plates arrive, I discreetly open it up on my lap and chow down! If you are a G-free guy, wear a jacket with roomy pockets, or find a good gal to throw some snacks in her bag.

Tip 3: Beware the influence of alcohol! Tips 1 and 2 will also equip you to avoid the many glutenous temptations that will be awaiting you at the wedding, especially if you drink alcohol. Anyone who has ever been on a diet—any diet—knows how this works: Have a couple of drinks, and all self-discipline goes out the window. Within seconds, you are right at the front of that buffet line.

Tip 4: Put your wingman to work. When I know my gluten alarm is about to be deactivated, I always make sure Tim is right next to me to prevent me from making a mistake I will spend the next week regret-ting. If you can't trust your own judgment in overamped, or overserved social situations, engage a gluten guard.

You could always just take the cookie and put it in your bag. Say, "Thank you *so* much! I cannot wait to give this to my husband/wife/boyfriend/roommate/kids—they will absolutely love it!" You'd be surprised by how well this one works! I have quite a few other methods that I use to rescue myself from awkward social situations—they are all worth trying out:

The swap: Try the old buddy-swap system again. Accept the treat, then sneakily pass it to your wingman when no one is looking. Practically foolproof!

The pawn: Accept the food, then gaze around the room in search of someone who looks hungry for seconds. Walk right up to that person and say, "This has your name written all over it!" Instead of offending anyone, you might just make a new friend!

The drop: If all else fails, you take the cookie and oopsie! You are just so clumsy, it's unforgivable! No, no, you couldn't *possibly* have another…

The pop: Take the cookie, and pop it right in your friend's mouth, exclaiming, "Oh, my—you have to taste this! Have you ever tried anything more delicious in your life?!" It's best to warn your buddy ahead of time that this might happen, *prior* to your little sabotage move.

G-Free Party Pack Favorites

Get into the habit of bringing your own drinks to any party. Here are some of my favorite on-the-go beverages that will guarantee you have a good time wherever you go!

BYOB!

Yes, there *are* G-free drinks you can bring to a party, more and more every year. These party-friendly beverages are all G-free.

Wine and champagne: In its pure form, wine is gluten-free, but to stay on the safe side, you should still contact the manufacturer to ensure that no glutenous additives have crept in along the way. Also check that the wine has been stored in gluten-free barrels—it sounds strange, I know, but it pays to be cautious! The same goes for champagne: It is almost always G-free. Wine coolers are *not* gluten-free, however, as they generally contain barley malt.

Gluten-free spirits: There's some debate over whether the grains are removed from alcoholic spirits in the distillation process. Luckily, there are some great—and totally safe—potato vodkas out there. My favorite is Chopin Vodka (www.chopinvodka.com). Japanese sake is also usually gluten-free in its pure form, but do check because sometimes cheap fillers are used to cut costs. Tequila, if free of additives, comes from the blue agave plant and should be G-free.

Gluten-free beers: Most beer is made from barley—a major no-no for anyone with a gluten sensitivity. But more and more companies are making celiac-friendly, G-free beers out of buckwheat, sorghum, millet, and rice. Every year, it seems like a new and delicious G-free beer hits the shelf of my local supermarket. Here are a few of my favorites:

- Bard's Tale Beer (www.bardsbeer.com).
- Lakefront Brewery (www.lakefrontbrewery.com).
- Ramapo Valley Brewery (http://ramapovalleybrewery.com).
- Redbridge Beer (www.redbridgebeer.com) was unveiled by Anheuser-Busch in 2006.
- Sprecher Brewery (www.sprecherbrewery.com).
- Microbreweries: Many local companies are responding to the call for a wider selection of gluten-free beers and offering beers safe for celiacs.

Action Checklist
- Whenever you accept an invitation, you should weigh the pros and cons of telling your host about your allergy.
- Buddy up with your party companion to protect yourself against gluten.
- Do not let peer pressure eclipse health considerations. A true friend will understand why you are declining a food.
- Be on guard around alcoholic beverages. They have a funny way of blunting your G-free resolve.
- To prevent late-night crises, pack snacks before leaving the house.

Out on the Town

The average American eats 4.2 meals a week away from home. For people with celiac disease, however, dining out in a restaurant can be stressful, and even scary. According to a recent Columbia University study of the impact of the gluten-free diet on quality of life, a whopping 86 percent of the respondents with celiac disease said that eating in restaurants created difficulties. And a larger study by the University of Ottawa found that over half of the celiac families surveyed avoided restaurants all or most of the time.

Does this mean you are doomed never to eat out again?

Not at *all!*

If you take the right precautions, you can enjoy eating out without endangering your health. As more and more people get diagnosed with celiac disease, more and more restaurants are offering gluten-free menu options, and they're also doing a better job of teaching their staff about the special requirements of G-free dieters. Every day, it becomes easier to dine out minus the fear of food.

Unfortunately, we still have a long way to go, and many restaurants are not that savvy when it comes to the G-free diet. Until the rest of the world catches on, you will need to master a few important rules before hitting the restaurant circuit. I have to warn you that the learning curve can be steep—for both you and the restaurants.

But the bottom line is that there is absolutely no reason to shut yourself into your kitchen for the rest of your life. With the right attitude and a little planning, you will not have to gamble with your body every time you walk into a restaurant.

Restaurant Etiquette

Before diagnosing myself with celiac disease, in addition to my unbearably painful symptoms, I felt hungry *all the time*. I later found out that many undiagnosed celiacs relate to this experience. It makes perfect sense: After all, when you are not absorbing any nutrients, how can you ever expect to feel full?

In my case, I would go without eating for extended periods of time because I had such acute stomach pains. Then, when I did feel well enough to eat, I'd go absolutely crazy, wildly stuffing my face in the hopes of finally feeling full. Even eating an entire tub of peanut butter in one sitting did not give me the feeling of satiety I so desperately craved.

Still, I was determined to get there, and in the early stages of my self-diagnosis, soon after I got back from Australia, Tim and I went out to a diner outside Boston. At the time, I had just begun removing wheat from my diet—I didn't yet know I couldn't eat any gluten—and I still was in pain most waking hours. But I was also feeling optimistic about the possibility of *finally* figuring out what was wrong with my body.

Tim and I, still in the early stages of dating, slid into the booth, and I ordered a regular omelet. "No toast, please," I added—and that was it. No details, no explanation, just "No toast, please."

When in Doubt: Plain over Pain!

The most important rule of eating outside your home is—Plain over Pain! This does not only apply to restaurant situations. When eating in a place where you are not certain of food preparation or ingredients—e.g., a restaurant, or hotel, or conference center—*always* pick completely plain food over complete pain in your abdomen.

When you step out of your comfort zone, the potential for pain is everywhere—your chicken might be premarinated in a bulk marinade that contains soy sauce, or some exotically named thickening agent that you have never heard of, or the seasoning used on your steak might come from a bulk bin with gluten added to unclump it. If you have any unresolved questions about the menu, play it safe. Choose the simplest food on the menu, and make sure that it's cooked on its own, with no potentially contaminated sauces or seasonings. You might feel boring tonight, but trust me, you will *not* regret the decision come tomorrow morning.

A few minutes later, my plate came out, with two buttery pieces of toast leaning right on top of the eggs. So what did I do? I burst into tears right there in the middle of the diner. So much for our breakfast date! Surprisingly, he asked me out again after that little meltdown—and has been a huge ally in my restaurant battles ever since!

I look back on this experience frequently, because it taught me several important lessons about navigating restaurants on the G-free diet.

One: Always take stock of *where* you are eating. I mean, really—have you ever heard of a diner that does not serve toast with every item on the menu?

Two: You have a responsibility to explain yourself, and make absolutely certain that you are heard and understood. While I thought I was getting a G-free meal, I was lazy when placing my order. How could I expect the waitress to read my mind and guess that my "No toast, please" request was the opposite of casual?

Three: If your waiter isn't writing down your instructions, or is giving you any other indicator that your message isn't getting through, you're probably better off going hungry.

The final lesson: People have good hearts, and generally want to help you. Make sure you give them that opportunity by telling them exactly *what* you need, and *why* you need it.

Tip 1: Do Your Work ahead of Time

I know, I know: You might feel a little embarrassed or uncomfortable at first, or just plain tired of explaining your condition a hundred times a day. But even if it sounds like a major hassle, I promise you a little advance preparation will pay off.

Call up the restaurant on the day you are planning to dine there, preferably in a slow hour between meal services. Talk to the hostess about your gluten allergy and discuss gluten-free items on the menu. If the restaurant seems unwilling to accommodate you—although I find this is rarely the case—you will probably get the hint on the phone. It's much better to discover this resistance in advance, when you still have time to change your plans.

Restaurant Tip

Do not walk into a restaurant forty minutes before the kitchen is closing and expect a G-free meal. If your dinner reservations are late at night, then call well in advance and give the chef time to make arrangements for your meal. Be as respectful of those creating your meal as you want them to be of your sensitivities!

You can also get good insights from visiting the restaurant's Web site. You can usually examine the menu online and determine the range of options available to you. The more research you do in advance, the more you will be able to relax and enjoy yourself in the moment. And wouldn't you rather focus on joking with your kids, or catching up with a college roommate you have not seen in three years? That's what I thought.

Tip 2: When You Get to the Restaurant, Ask to Speak to the Manager

This is another better-safe-than-sorry technique that I highly recommend, especially on your first trip to any restaurant. Sometimes, servers might be new on the job and relatively inexperienced, or they might be juggling two dozen tables the moment you show up. It's your job to make sure that the staff understands your gluten-free diet, and the best way to do that is to talk to the manager.

In my waitressing days, whenever a customer told me about a food allergy, I'd always call my manager over anyway, without being asked. I didn't want to hurt anybody, and I knew that my manager was more experienced and better equipped to handle the situation. That's still a good operating assumption. The vast majority of restaurant managers know all about celiac disease, and they also have

---

Better Safe Than Sorry: Deep-Fried Foods

Never order fried foods without making sure that they haven't been breaded in flour, or cooked in a deep fryer where flour is used. At a Mexican restaurant, you should always ask if the chip fryer is reserved for corn chips only.

more at stake than members of the waitstaff. Count on the manager to inform the kitchen of your special dietary needs.

Tip 3: Don't Shoot the Messenger

Some more all-purpose advice, for the G-free and everyone else: You catch more bees with honey. If your order arrives messed up, don't lose your cool. I know that the waitstaff's just trying to do their job—and an incredibly difficult job at that (I know, I have been there). It's not just that they're working a million tables at the same time; it's that they don't actually have control over the food that's coming out of the kitchen. Most waiters are eager to help, so treat them as allies, not enemies.

Tip 4: Employ Some Power Phrases

Language is important, and often, the phrases you choose will affect how seriously people take your requests. If you leave it at "I am not eating gluten right now," then the waitress might not take careful notes on your order. Good luck getting a gluten-free meal. Remember my Boston diner story: Simply saying "No toast, please" is not *nearly* enough information.

If, on the other hand, you say, "I have celiac disease and cannot eat gluten," or "I have a severe allergy to gluten," chances are, the person taking your order will pay close attention. Phrases like "disease" and "severe allergy" are red flags in restaurant settings, and will most likely trigger the desired response. If you *still* feel like your waiter isn't taking you seriously, don't be afraid to amp up your language even more. "I will have to leave here in an ambulance if my food is touching anything with gluten" has been used in extreme circumstances.

Tip 5: Be Specific to Be Safe

Remember our golden rule: Plain over Pain. To ensure your meal won't hurt you, use words like "naked" and "dry" when placing your order. If the steak you're ordering normally comes with a butter sauce, you need to be *very* specific in asking for it dry. Say, for example, "I would like my steak naked. Just olive oil, salt and pepper, nothing else, please. It has to be made in a clean pan with nothing else in it." Or: "Please do not put any bread on the same plate as my steak. I have celiac disease, so if bread touches any food that I eat, I will get incredibly sick on the spot."

One trick that I find works really well: Tell your waiter *exactly* what your plate should look like. Say, "I would like a plate with *just* my hard-boiled eggs on it, nothing else." Or if I am splitting my dinner with Grace, I will ask to have each separate component of the meal put on a separate plate. "Please put the chicken on one plate and that's it," I will say. "Please put the salad on another plate, and the mashed potatoes on a third plate—so that's three plates total." (I know…they must love me!!!!) *Always leave a generous tip.*

Put Your Needs on Paper

Best bet: Make it official! Writing down your dietary requirements ahead of time can save time and hassle in a restaurant setting. It can also be a favor to the people preparing your meal. Recently, a few minutes after I handed the waiter my card, the chef actually came out of the kitchen to thank me: "I've heard of celiac disease, but sometimes, people seem to assume that I am a doctor. But I am not; I am a chef." He told me that the details on my card really helped him craft a meal for me that would be both safe and delicious. So trust me—these cards work! Don't leave home without one. There's one included at the back of this book for your convenience.

By requesting separate plates for each dish, you won't have to worry about the gluten-containing mashed potatoes coming into contact with your gluten-free chicken.

Tip 6: BYO Seasoning—Or Whatever Else You'd Like

Less than thrilled about that plain-and-dry slab of meat placed in front of you? Well, you can do what I often do: Bring your own seasoning! Before leaving home, prepare a small container of your favorite G-free ketchup or soy sauce or salad dressing. I often stash some Amy's Honey Mustard in my purse, just because I want my meal to have a little zest.

Sometimes, I will bring more than just a little seasoning to a restaurant—I will bring my entire meal! It helps that I am the mother of young kids: Moms can get away with just about anything in restaurants, as far as I can tell. I can pretty much carry my own food into a restaurant, camouflage it as my kids', then pretend I am "snacking" on it while actually eating the whole thing myself! No explanations, and no one ever blinks an eye.

Obviously, neither of these solutions is ideal: I hope that one day

---

Better Safe Than Sorry: Eggs

A plate of eggs sounds dependably gluten-free, right? Not so fast: Some popular restaurants and pancake chains add a little pancake batter to the eggs to give them a lighter, fluffier appearance. Also, eggs are often prepared in the same kitchen—sometimes the same pan—as pancakes or other baked goods, which poses another contamination risk. Or a cook might use a contaminated stick of butter, or a nonstick spray with grain alcohol. To protect yourself from these pitfalls, you should always check before ordering eggs.

I will no longer have to pack up my own food when going out to eat. Who knows—maybe in twenty years, I will laugh when I remember all those nights that I took my honey mustard dressing along, prayed the Ziploc commercials were telling the truth and that my "sneaky flavor" wouldn't explode in my favorite bag on the way to the restaurant. Until that time comes, you just have to get used to making these minor adjustments.

Tip 7: Don't Take a Bite Just to Be Polite ... Redux

Same rule applies to restaurants as to social situations: You are the customer, and you are paying to enjoy yourself—try not to lose sight of that fact. If you are not bold enough to send your meal back if you suspect contamination, you will pay for your timidity in stomach cramps later. If your plate contains even a trace of gluten, never hesitate to send it back—and do not accept half-measures. Additionally, if you point out to your server that your meat is touching a piece of bread, sometimes someone trying to help will just toss the bread and send out the same contaminated plate a second time. Or if your salad is covered in croutons, some restaurants will just pick off the offending breadcrumbs and send out the exact same salad again.

Buffet: No Way!!!!

Tongs travel. A lot. Think about it: The tongs that were in your salad also touched many other substances at some point. The typical restaurant buffet line is a breeding ground for cross-contamination. I would avoid these types of settings, or request that your meal be made from scratch in the kitchen. You want to be able to talk with the person preparing your food.

Better Safe Than Sorry: Ice Cream

While some ice cream that you can buy at the store is naturally gluten-free, ice cream scoops are often contaminated by constant contact with gluten-containing ice cream cones, flavors, and toppings (for example, cookie dough, pretzels, and cookies-and-cream). As always, you should study the list of ingredients and call the company before making the plunge. Dove Dark Chocolate Ice Cream Bars are a safe bet. (Dove has a wonderful policy of declaring gluten on the labels of all its products, which has earned the loyalty of many a celiac!) Frozen yogurts are not all gluten-free, as they often contain a modi-fied food starch, though Red Mango frozen yogurt—which I love—is. Pinkberry yogurt and Skinny Cow ice cream bars are also gluten-free.

Ice cream that comes out of a machine is generally less of a con-tamination risk, but beware those big tubs that have been sitting open all day. You can only really be positive that your ice cream is uncon-taminated if you ask the server to open a new tub and use a clean scoop for you...Making this request can often seem like more trouble than it's worth, but take my word on this one: When you have scored a G-free cup of dessert, you will have no regrets.

And if eating out of a cup does not cut it, Barkat makes wonderful G-free ice cream cones, which you can buy at the Gluten-Free Mall (www.glutenfreemall.com). The regular Barkat cones also contain no eggs, nuts, or dairy, so they're safe for people with a range of food allergies.

Forewarned is forearmed! Mark the contaminated food so you will be sure to recognize it a second time. I suggest that you cut your meat in half; douse that salad with dressing and *then* send it back. Whether you carve your initials into a burger or throw a bottle of ketchup all over the salad prior to bidding it farewell, make certain that the food that comes back to you is new and uncontaminated. You should also ask for new utensils with the new plate of food.

Deciphering the Menu: The G-Free Detective

Early on, you should familiarize yourself with common menu terms that translate to "gluten, gluten, gluten"! Be on the lookout for all these terms, most of which are no-nos in any language.

Au gratin: Au gratin describes a dish cooked with a topping of bread crumbs and sometimes butter or grated cheese as well.

Battered: A "battered" food has usually been slathered in a coating of wheat flour, eggs, and milk.

Béchamel: This white sauce, which is common in French cuisine, is made by thickening milk with wheat flour and butter.

Beurre manié: Beurre manié, a paste made of flour and butter, is used to thicken sauces.

Bisque: A smooth, creamy shellfish soup that's often thickened with flour.

Breaded: This one's pretty easy to decipher: Breaded equals breadcrumbs equals gluten. The term "coated" is often a synonym for "breaded," so watch out for that one, too.

Cordon bleu: Chicken cordon bleu (there's also veal cordon bleu) is chicken coated in breadcrumbs.

Croquette: A croquette is a puree of vegetables, seafood, or cheese that has been coated in breadcrumbs, then deep-fried or sautéed.

Croutons: Croutons are cubed pieces of bread, lightly baked or fried, often sprinkled over salads and soups. Try making your own G-free variations!

Crusted: The word "crusted" (and "encrusted," too) refers to a food that has been coated with flour or breadcrumbs.

Demi-glace: This rich, concentrated stock almost always contains flour.

Dredged: Dragged through flour, cornmeal, or breadcrumbs.

Dumplings: Dumplings are usually made out of wheat flour.

Dusted: This word almost always indicates the presence of flour.

En croûte: An "en croûte" food has been baked in pastry crust.

Espagnole: Espagnole sauce has almost always been thickened with flour.

Farfel: A soup garnish made of finely chopped or minced noodle dough.

Filo: Filo, or phyllo, is a flaky, paper-thin pastry made from wheat flour.

Fricassée: A stew of meat or poultry in gravy, usually thickened with flour.

Fritter: Food that has been dipped in a flour-containing batter and then fried.

Gnocchi: A variation on traditional Italian pasta, gnocchi are dense dumplings made from a paste of flour, potatoes, and eggs.

Gravy: Gravy is a general term for a range of sauces, which are usually made from meat juices and often thickened with flour.

Marinade: A marinade might contain soy sauce or other glutenous ingredients.

Meunière: A French preparation that usually involves dusting meat with flour and then sautéing it in butter.

Milanaise: An Italian preparation that involves dipping meat in egg and breadcrumbs, then frying it in butter.

Raspings: Raspings are finely ground breadcrumbs.

Roux: Roux is a paste of butter (or some other fat) and flour used to thicken sauces and soups.

Scallopini: Thin-sliced meat usually coated with flour and fried.

Soufflé: A fluffy dish that usually contains flour.

Soy sauce: Most soy sauces contain roasted wheat or barley. You might have to bring your own along.

Streusel: A crumbly dessert component that is made from flour, butter, sugar, and spices.

Teriyaki sauce: Contains soy sauce.

Tempura: A Japanese method of frying foods in a flour-based batter. Some Japanese restaurants use rice flour for a lighter texture, but you should assume the opposite and check with the kitchen before ordering.

Safe International Bets

Most Indian restaurants use very little gluten. Vietnamese restaurants are also a fairly safe bet. You can also find good options at many Mexican restaurants—just make sure your corn tortillas never touch the flour ones or the steam press. Have them microwaved separately. If you are going out for Japanese or Chinese food, you might want to bring your own wheat-free tamari.

Velouté: Sauce thickened with flour.

Welsh rarebit: Cheese sauce made with ale or beer and served over toast or crackers.

Ordering In

A word of warning here: When you order food in, you might be creating stomach problems for yourself. The restaurant's level of accountability is much lower when the customer isn't sitting right there, detailing how the meal should be prepared. Restaurants have much more of an incentive to get things right when you are on-site. Your order could easily be mixed up with someone else's, or your specific instructions lost in translation over the phone. Rather than take these chances, I suggest keeping some G-free frozen options on hand for those nights when your family members feel like getting food delivered. Pop in your meal a few minutes after you place the order, and your meal will be ready at the same time the food reaches your door.

Favorite Restaurants

Over time, you will develop your own loyalties to restaurants in your area—staffs that go out of their way to accommodate you, or cuisines that naturally use very little gluten. In New York, I love Sambuca (www.sambucanyc.com), because it has a separate gluten-free kitchen. Their chocolate brownie is the best! I am also a huge fan of Slice (www.sliceperfect.com), a pizza place that caters to all different diets: They have G-free, wheat-free, and regular pizza—all prepared in separate dedicated ovens. I cannot tell you how wonderful it is to bite into a delicious slice of pizza and know that I won't be sick the next day! And I can't forget Babycakes NYC (www.babycakesnyc.com)…The best of G-free and sweet as can be! GROM in New York City also makes delicious (and frequently G-free) Italian gelatos. Check the Web site for details.

In addition to your own local favorites, you can rely on a number of national chains for safe, delicious, G-free meals out. There's nothing like washing up in a new city and knowing that you will be able to get a good meal! Many of these restaurants even offer downloadable gluten-free menus that you can study (or memorize!) in advance:

- Austin Grill (www.austingrill.com).
- Blue Ginger (www.ming.com/blueginger): Ming Tsai's wonderful restaurant in the Boston suburbs goes to great lengths to cater to people with all sorts of food allergies.
- Bonefish Grill (Bonefishgrill.com/pdf/bfg_menu_gf.pdf).
- Boston Market (www.bostonmarket.com/restaurant?page =allergens): We love stopping here with the kids. Always ask your server to put on new gloves to avoid cross-contamination!
- Carrabba's Italian Grill (www.carrabbas.com/menu/pdf/ GFMenu.pdf).
- Chick-fil-A (www.chick-fil-a.com/gluten.asp 800 cfa-2040).
- Chili's (www.chilis.com) has a list of gluten-free menu items that changes every month.
- Chipotle (www.chiplote.com): I order a burrito bowl with no cheese or lettuce. Have them change their gloves before they prepare your bowl—the people at Chipotle are great about that.
- Dairy Queen (www.dairyqueen.com/us-en/eats-and-treats/

gluten-free-products/): If we see one, we stop! It's a family addiction. I would stay away from the Blizzards, however—you cannot guarantee that those mixing tins are entirely free of gluten. I stick with the old-school chocolate-vanilla swirl, or a prepackaged bar.

- Denny's (www.dennys.com/en/page.asp?PID=1&ID=23).
- Don Pablo's (www.donpablos.com): I ate here all the time when Tim was on the Redskins. I would recommend talking to the manager when you arrive to make sure that the chips are the only items on the fryer, and that the corn tortillas stay far away from the general steamer.
- Jamba Juice (www.jambajuice.com/what/faq/html): Though most smoothies are G-free, many of the supplements are not, so I will not order a smoothie unless I can get into the kitchen and clean out the blender myself.
- Legal Seafoods (www.legalseafoods.com): This place makes a great dinner after a long day of shopping at the mall. As always, make sure that your veggies are boiled in fresh water (no pasta water!) and talk to the manager about your allergy before sitting down.
- Maggiano's (www.maggianos.com): Take the same precautions at Maggiano's. I love this place so much that I had my bachelorette party here in Boston!
- McDonald's (www.mcdonalds.com): The fries are *not* G-free, as they contain wheat and wheat derivatives.
- Mitchell's Fish Market (www.mitchellsfishmarket.com).
- Outback Steakhouse (www.outback.com/pirmenu/pdf/glu tenfree.pdf): Check to make sure that the salad has no citric acid, which can set off some celiac stomachs. Otherwise, a great G-free menu!
- Pei Wei Asian Diner (www.peiwei.com/glutenfreeMenu.jsp).
- P.F. Chang's (www.pfchangs.com/cuisine/menu_spec.jsp): I love, love, *love* P.F. Chang's, which has a separate G-free menu, and they even serve their G-free options on special plates, so

you know your message got through! I wish more restaurants would do this—it makes me feel so much safer. Tim and Grace always order the lettuce wraps with me, so we can all eat the same appetizer. The only problem with the rest of the meal is that you have to defend your plate from everyone else's forks!

- Red Lobster (www.redlobster.com).
- Subway (www.subway.com/applications/NutritionInfo/index .aspx).
- Taco Del Mar (www.tacodelmar.com/food/gluten.html).
- Texas Roadhouse (www.texasroadhouse.com).
- Wendy's (www.wendys.com/food/pdf/us/gluten_free_list.pdf): Another family favorite. I always order a large chili straight up, a plain baked potato, and a medium chocolate Frosty. (Sometimes I order a large, but that's a napper...meaning I have to take a nap immediately afterward.) It's always a quiet ride home when we all have our straws in our mouths and are inhaling our Frostys. I avoid anything put on the grill—not that I mind, since the Frosty is all that matters!
- Aquagrill (www.aquagrill.com) in New York also makes it very easy to dine out without fear of being glutened.

Action Checklist

- Plain over Pain is the Number 1 rule to live by when venturing out of your house to eat.
- You have an obligation to tell servers all the information necessary to provide a safe meal for you, in as much detail as possible.
- Research safe options *before* leaving home. You will have more fun that way.
- Be polite, and tip generously.
- Avoid buffets and salad bars, and be wary of egg dishes and ice cream scoopers.
- When sending food back, mark it so you know the same piece isn't coming back to you.
- Memorize menu terms that might translate to gluten.

11

Traveling G-Free

Vacation is supposed to be a time of total relaxation, when you can put all the hassles of your day-to-day existence on hold, if just for a few glorious days. No more alarm clock, or job, or household chores to cramp your style. The time is yours to enjoy. Exhale.

There is just one catch! Your G-free diet is a 365-days-a-year commitment, and straying from it can be particularly dangerous when you are far from home. Though it is slightly more complicated to obtain safe food when on the road for a period of time, it is by no means impossible. Sticking to the core playbook that gets you through dinner parties and weddings healthy and happy will be your best strategy. Once the destination is set, your flight, train, or bus booked, hotel reserved, car rented, tickets confirmed, and your research done ahead of time to protect your body, you will be in for the trip of a lifetime. The more work you do at home, the better time you will have away!

Basic Travel Tips

Pack as many high-protein snacks as you can cram into your suitcase. Whether you are traveling across the state or across several oceans, you should always bring along plenty of protein bars and any other prepackaged comfort foods. I never go *anywhere* without a large supply of nuts, seeds, and my trusty protein bars. Portable forms of protein will give you much-needed energy for long days on your feet—it sure beats swooning from hunger while standing in line at the Magic Kingdom! If your trip is a long one, and there is little or no room for the stash of goodies, pack enough to get you through the first few days, then ship the rest to your destination. You should also bring all the soaps and shampoos that you normally use at home—do not count on a hotel (or a friend's guest bathroom) to stock reliably G-free beauty products.

Be open about your dietary needs. Whether you are staying at a hotel or in a relative's guest room, make sure the people in charge know all about your diet. Call your hotel, or your host, well in advance of your arrival. Even if you are only staying somewhere for a few nights, you need to specify exactly what you can and can't eat. Keep asking questions until you are satisfied with the answers. (I used to eat hard-boiled eggs at the hotel breakfast bar until I realized they were cooked in the same pot used to make pasta—it wasn't until I asked the chef that I figured out what was going on.) To make sure everything that passes your lips is safe, have these conversations before you arrive, the day you get there, and (if necessary) prior to every subsequent meal.

Research local restaurants and stores. Before leaving on your trip, look up celiac-friendly restaurants in the area. If there are no local restaurants *or* chains with G-free menus (like Outback Steakhouse, Wendy's, or P.F. Chang's), make your dinner reservations ahead of

time and specify your need for G-free food. You could also consider faxing them your G-free needs. Locate a nearby health food
store where you can get your fix of gluten-free goodies. You can ask
your hotel for advice on this front. As you would do when preparing for a night out in your town, try connecting with the restaurant manager before you show up to make sure you will be taken
care of.

Shop upon arrival. Lots of people head straight for the tourist
landmarks when they arrive at a new place. Not in my case!—I bee-
line for the local grocery store! Whatever your destination, you will
be able to stock up on safe, delicious foods like fruits, nuts, rai-
sins, and candies. Ask the hotel ahead of time for a minifridge and
microwave, and let them know about your allergy. If you are staying in a place where you can make your own food—a friend's house
or a rental—ensure that all food prep areas are sanitized and safe.
Wash all appliances, utensils, and surfaces. Before making your
food, cover baking sheets and toaster oven bottoms with foil. If you
are staying somewhere for an extended period, you should consider
bringing along your own small pot, or buying one at the local store.
I don't trust communal pots and pans, no matter how many times
they've gone through the dishwasher—that pasta residue can be
awfully stubborn.

SURVIVAL GUIDE: THE G-FREE HOUSEGUEST

Crashing at a friend or relative's place? Then make absolutely certain the people hosting you understand (and respect!) your diet.
Before your visit, have an open conversation with your hosts about
what you can and cannot eat. Load up your suitcase with safe
foods—and bring enough for everyone to sample! I also recommend
stopping off at the grocery store for some safe snacks and frozen
foods to keep on hand for the duration of your stay. If you are visiting someone long term, you might want to go online and get some

of your favorite G-free staples shipped to your hosts: G-free pastas, some favorite cookies, or chips.

If your hosts are overwhelmed by these requests, assure them that you are a pro at determining foods that might make you sick. Let them know that you can *always* find something to eat, and that you will be coming with some great treats that you are excited to share!

Dealing with the Type A, love-you-so-much-I-am-going-to-make-everything-I-make-best-gluten-free-just-for-you host can be a bit trickier. Yes, your superhuman hostess *is* going to have an apple strudel waiting for you. In fact, she has made two—there's another in the freezer for tomorrow night, to be eaten right after the extraspecial gluten-free potpie she has concocted.

First off, never underestimate the incredible kindness of these efforts. What a great friend! That said, you still have a responsibility to your body and your health, so if you feel comfortable enough, ask, with *full* excitement and curiosity, exactly how she made it. Say that you want to "try to do it at home." (This is my celiac code for: Tell me every single ingredient, and every single step of the cooking process, and while you are at it, show me all the bottles—so I can be *sure* that it really is G-free.)

You can pick up a lot of clues from hearing about the process, so it helps to ask these questions right away, before taking your first bite. I remember once I asked a friend how she made G-free corn muffins only *after* eating one, only to find out that the muffin pan was "dusted with flour," my host's "little secret to keep them from sticking." The look on my face said it all, and my host was devastated. "I thought there just couldn't be gluten *in* the recipe!" she cried. "I figured a little flour on the pan would be fine. I feel awful!" She really did. But I felt worse!

Keep in mind: Graciousness is your Number 1 duty as a houseguest, and keeping yourself healthy should in *no* way conflict with this duty. While you do want to educate your hosts about your diet, you don't want to dictate what *they* eat, or make them feel awkward

---

Your G-Free Houseguest

If you are about to host a G-free houseguest, your first duty should be to talk to your guest about which foods (and cooking styles) cause problems. An open dialogue will dramatically lower the risk of accidents or awkwardness—I have no doubt that your houseguest will be relieved to talk openly about what the G-free diet entails! I offer some tips in the next chapter about how to live with a G-freer; you can apply many of the same guidelines to temporary cohabitation.

---

about enjoying their favorite foods. If your hosts always order pizza on Tuesday nights, encourage that tradition to continue while you are in town—just pop your own G-free frozen meal in the microwave and join in the fun!

SURVIVAL GUIDE: THE G-FREE GLOBETROTTER

Sticking to your G-free diet in foreign countries isn't as tricky as you might think. In fact, in many places, it's actually *easier* to avoid gluten than it is here in the States. Quite a few countries—Italy, Australia, Finland, to name just a few—are decades ahead of us when it comes to labeling allergen-containing foods. Restaurants in these countries are also better educated about celiac disease and wheat allergies.

Still, whenever you travel to a country where English isn't the first language, you should *always* bring along a translated version of your G-free card to show waiters and chefs. If you are supermotivated, you might even want to memorize the words for "celiac" or "gluten" in the language of the country you are visiting. And while you are packing, flip through *Let's Eat Out! Your Passport to Living Gluten and Allergy Free* for more specific advice on country-by-country cooking techniques and ingredients.

As you'd do on any trip away from home, be sure to educate your hotel's staff (or your hosts) before you roll into town. E-mail a list of prohibited foods if you can. A quick long-distance exchange will be a courtesy for your hosts, and a potential lifesaver for you. And don't forget to pack (or ship) plenty of prepackaged foods to keep you going strong throughout the trip. The last place you want to be while in Italy or Spain is in the bathroom of your hotel room every twenty minutes!

SURVIVAL GUIDE: THE G-FREE ROAD-TRIPPER

Before filling up your tank and packing up your trunk, go online and research gluten-free options at roadside fast-food restaurants in the area you will be visiting. Print out their menus and ingredient lists (for more information, see pages 134–37). Stash this material in your glove compartment for easy access. For the gung-ho G-freer: Get those menus in plastic sleeves and make them for keeps! Over the next few days, these printouts will be as essential to you as highway maps. Think about it: When you pull into a rest stop with a Wendy's or a TCBY, you are not going to have time to call customer service right then. You also probably won't have Internet access to do your sleuthing online. You need to know what exactly you can and can't eat *before* hitting the open road. There's nothing worse (for you *or* your travel companions) than falling ill when you are trapped in a car for hours on end. And as always, pack plenty of your own snacks for a road trip, so that if you happen to stop at a gas station with a limited selection of foods, you won't feel left out when everybody else loads up on treats.

The iPhone has a gluten-free restaurant card application, and many other mobile phones can help guide you to G-free eating on the road.

Action Checklist

- A trip is really no different from a night out in a restaurant: It's all about advance planning.
- Research everything thoroughly, and pack enough protein bars and snacks to get you through the first few days away from home.
- Take your G-free dining card with you everywhere you go. If you are traveling to a foreign country, bring a translated version.
- Tell your host, or your hotel, about your allergy to minimize the risk of trouble.

12

G-Free Kids

The consequences of chronic malnutrition are never more serious than in early childhood, when the body is developing at an incredibly fast rate. Improper nutrition in early childhood can impair children's growth and many aspects of their development, including their ability to concentrate and to learn.

Why am I telling you this? Because undiagnosed celiac disease is becoming a real health crisis among children today. Ranked as the most common chronic childhood disease, celiac disease might affect as many as 1 in 80 children worldwide. The earlier children are diagnosed with the disorder, the better their long-term prognosis.

Stage I: Diagnosing Your Child

Only a doctor can diagnose your child with celiac disease or a serious gluten intolerance, but only *you* can know when your child is acting abnormally.

STEP 1: BE VIGILANT

Celiac disease is a genetic disorder, which means that your child is either predisposed to have it or not. If you or your partner—or any of your first-degree relatives—has celiac disease, then you need to be supervigilant, even in the earliest months of your child's life. Your child's chances of having the condition are higher than average: 1 in 22 if a parent or sibling has celiac disease. You should also talk to your doctor about an appropriate food introduction schedule. You might be told to introduce gluten a little later if you fear some sensitivity.

Early on in your child's life, you are already watching every movement so closely, charting each and every developmental milestone. Look out for any telltale signs and symptoms. If you have a two-year-old who is lethargic all the time (and anyone who has ever dealt with a toddler knows that lethargy is *not* usually an issue!), then don't ignore those signs. A low weight percentile, poor coloring, and gastrointestinal complaints could all point to a larger problem. Could it be celiac disease? Only a doctor can tell you for certain.

No matter what, you should trust your intuition, and always, always consult your pediatrician about any concerns you may have. It's helpful to take thorough, day-by-day notes on your child's behavior, so that you can give your doctor the information necessary to move forward. Children are not always capable of articulating their distress, which can complicate the diagnostic process all the more. A parent's careful observations can make all the difference in the world.

STEP 2: GET TESTED

If you continue to track symptoms that your doctor cannot explain, your next step should be to get your child tested. You should *only* do this if your child's behavior indicates that there might be a problem. The blood tests and, even more so, the endoscopic biopsy are invasive procedures, not to be taken lightly.

One Mother's Story

Kathy Burger's daughter, Katie, was diagnosed at the age of 2 1/2.

From the time that Katie was about six or nine months old, she had chronic sinusitis, so she was constantly on antibiotics. And as most parents know, when small children are on antibiotics, they have tummy issues, so we assumed that antibiotics were responsible for Katie's constant diarrhea and bellyaches. Finally, when Katie was about twenty-two months old, she had surgery to unblock one of her nasal passages. After the surgery, she was no longer on antibiotics, but the bellyaches didn't stop. That was when I knew something wasn't right. Even after we'd eliminated the other issue, she still had these problems. When I talked to my pediatrician, she told me that Katie had a condition called "toddler's diarrhea," which was comparable to IBS in an adult and no big deal. So I let it go for a while, but—call it mother's intuition—I still kept saying to my husband: "Something's not right." I was changing Katie's diaper fifteen to twenty times a day. It was unbelievable. And it was very small amounts, so the doctors kept saying it was a control thing—that she wouldn't "let" herself go. And it's hard, because you kind of take what the doctors say as the truth—you believe them!

Still, I just knew something wasn't right. Aside from the diarrhea, Katie would lie on the floor and just moan, when other kids her age were playing. She was also very different at home than she was anywhere else. At home, she was social, and talkative, and loving; she was receptive to hugs and kisses. But outside of our house, she was a totally different child. She wouldn't talk to people. She was not receptive to any kind of attention. Sometimes she could be nasty and rude, even to her grandparents or her cousins. That was very

(*continued*)

frustrating for my husband and me—the fact that no one got to see the real Katie.

Throughout all of this, she never complained. She was very verbal; she spoke at age one, so it wasn't that she couldn't complain. But she never did. She didn't want to eat. She would often say, "I don't want to eat. I don't feel like eating." She had always been a picky eater—she still is—and at one point, she just stopped eating all the staple kid-friendly foods, like macaroni and cheese, chicken nuggets, and pizza, foods she had always loved before. And I really think it was because everything made her feel sick, but she never verbalized that to us. I don't know if she fully made the connection herself, because she could have said those words if she'd wanted to.

If I hadn't been so persistent, she wouldn't have been diagnosed. I finally insisted on seeing a specialist. When I told him our whole story, he was very impressed. He asked me if I had a medical background, and I said no. And this is something I recommend every parent do: I took notes constantly on Katie. From the time she was a baby and had continuing sinus infections, I wrote down all the medications she took, all the effects they had on her; I kept timelines. Nobody else knows your child like you do, especially if you are going to multiple doctors. My notes really helped this specialist get a better picture of what was going on in Katie's life. Based on that information, and a thorough exam—he did blood work and collected a stool sample—he was able to diagnose her with celiac disease. He looked at us and said, "This is wonderful news!" My husband and I had no idea what he meant: What was wonderful about having a disease? But what the doctor meant was that it was wonderful that we found out so early. And I believe that now, but I didn't at the time...

Katie was sitting in the office eating a bag of pretzels and the doctor said, "Okay, she can't eat that anymore." It was very abrupt. He gave us a big packet of information about the gluten-free diet, set us up with a nutritionist—and then basically sent us on our way. I cried

> the entire way home. I was depressed, and angry, and panicked. "Why me? Why her?" I kept thinking. "Why my baby girl?" I felt a real sense of loss, and sadness for her, and everything she was going to miss out on in life because of this disease.
>
> —*Kathy Burger*

STEP 3: WHAT NOW???

Having a child test positive for celiac disease will probably come as a major blow to you and your family, but do not despair: As at any stage of life, a gluten-free diet is usually all it takes to set the healing in motion. Yes, the diet does present challenges, but it is also a great opportunity to restore your child's health and happiness—a small price to pay in the larger scheme of things!

Stage II: Feeding Your Child

STEP 1: SHOP FOR KID-FRIENDLY FOOD

Hit the grocery store right away. Shop for basic foods that will please your kids without too much labor. Corn tortilla tacos or a G-free pasta salad make easy one-dish meals for the whole family. The most important thing to remember as you browse the aisles is that you *will* find food that your G-free kid can eat and enjoy—you just might have to look a little harder for it at first. Van's gluten-free waffles, Ian's gluten-free chicken nuggets, Pamela's gluten-free cookies and cake mixes are all safe, convenient, and guaranteed to bring a smile to your child's face.

STEP 2: DESIGN DAILY MENUS

Organizing what to feed your child in advance will help all of you adjust to this change in lifestyle. Ashley Koff, RD, has designed a sample kids' menu to give you some ideas:

Breakfast

Option 1: Plain yogurt sundae (look for one serving to equal about 15 grams total carbohydrate): Add banana slices and unsweetened coconut slivers and sprinkle some chopped nuts and cinnamon over the top.

Option 2: Rice or corn flakes with coconut and nuts and berries in a bowl with milk or milk replacement.

School Snack

Option 1: G-free waffle with almond butter and sliced strawberries and/or honey, folded in half.

Option 2: G-free rice-snap chips with almond butter and a side of canned pineapple.

Option 3: G-free cereal bar.

Lunch

Option 1: Lunchbox taco salad (corn tortilla chips, chopped/ground turkey, beans, guacamole, shredded cheese, salsa), fruit skewers on Popsicle sticks.

Option 2: G-free sandwich with G-free turkey (Applegate Farms or Hormel), Amy's honey mustard sauce, lettuce, and G-free cheese.

After-School Snack

Option 1: Sweet potato pudding or veggie sticks with hummus.

Option 2: Kozy Shack pudding.

Option 3: Cashews, strawberries.

Option 4: Pamela's cookie with milk.

Dinner

Chopped veggie salad with mozzarella cubes, chicken sausage, tingly fruit salad (berries and melon balls mixed with mint and honey, agave nectar, or sugar).

STEP 3: COOK AND BAKE TOGETHER

Right away, you should get your G-free kids in the kitchen. Baking with your G-free child is an important tool for teaching him to take ownership of his special diet. The more he knows, the more in control he is…and the more fun he can have with his food.

Surviving Birthday Parties

For us G-freers, birthday parties and other social events can be tricky at any age, but kids face particular difficulties. A little advance planning is the best way to keep your kid safe in a setting full of allergens. "I have a calendar with the birthdays of all the children in Katie's class," Kathy Burger told me when I asked how she coped with these situations. "I call the moms ahead of time and ask what they are bringing, and then I try to bring something comparable for Katie. She doesn't like to have attention drawn to the fact that she has celiac disease, so having a look-alike substitution really helps."

Kathy adopts a similar strategy at weekend birthday parties. "I keep a stash of chocolate and vanilla gluten-free cupcakes in my freezer," she said, "so whenever we're going to a birthday party, I call ahead and ask 'What kind of cake are you having?' I'm not trying to be a pain—I just want Katie's treat to look like everybody else's. As long as I have this control at this age," Kathy added, "I'm going to do everything I can to make her feel like everybody else. There's going to come a point where I don't have that, so I'm going to do everything I can now."

Whenever one of her nonceliac sons has a birthday party, Kathy will make two separate cakes. "Last year, my son wanted a *Star Wars* party, so I made a Death Star cake and a Lightsaber cake. The Death Star cake was regular, and the Lightsaber cake was gluten-free. That way, Katie can feel like she can have what everybody else is having."

Learn a few easy recipes that you can make together—this will really help your kids understand what goes into their food. When they get older, they will be grateful for these lessons, and perhaps less likely to rebel against their diets.

There are a number of G-free cookbooks aimed especially at kids, such as *Incredible Edible Gluten-Free Food for Kids: 150 Family Tested Recipes* by Sheri Sanderson. The *Wheat-Free Gluten-Free Cookbook for Kids and Busy Adults* by Connie Sarros also has some quick and easy recipes that you can try with your kids. Vanessa Maltin's *Beyond Rice Cakes: A Young Person's Guide to Cooking, Eating, and Living Gluten-Free* is targeted at college-age kids and young adults entering the world on their own for the first time.

Stage III: Empowering Your Child

Instilling good eating habits early in life is of paramount importance for *all* children. It is even more important if your child cannot tolerate one of the most ubiquitous of all foods. Early on, you need to remove any mystique that might surround the G-free diet. Start an ongoing dialogue about what your kids are eating and why.

STEP 1: ARM THEM WITH INFORMATION

Every parent knows that if there's anything kids like more than asking questions, it's getting answers. Kids *love* new information, and you should use their insatiable curiosity to your advantage. Kids are especially interested in any and all information that pertains to them personally. To the greatest extent possible, you should openly talk to your kids about what having an allergy means, and engage in constant question-and-answer sessions about food. Pick up the conversation when you are shopping at the grocery store, and when you are unpacking your groceries. Try to think of ways to make G-free living fun for your kids—like setting up a G-free scavenger hunt. Or you could get your child special G-free stickers to put on the special food…with a different color sticker for each sibling! Mabel's Labels are my standby—you can label everything with them.

STEP 2: FOCUS ON THE FUN

When teaching your kids about the G-free diet, always keep the information at a level that they can handle, and make it seem fun and exciting—more an adventure than an obligation. "Hey, guess what—we're going to talk about being G-free. The best part is that these cookies will not make you sick!!!"

If you keep the lines of communication open, your G-free kids will come to take pride in their diet. Make them feel special—in a good way. They shouldn't see their diet as a stigma or a punishment, but as a special thing that sets them apart. "Hey, you know what, there are certain foods that make your tummy sick—you remember how your tummy felt when you had that other food? Well, we have a really incredible, special brownie for you, and it will make you strong."

If your child seems embarrassed by having something "different," some would recommend not making a big deal out of the new version of the pancake or waffle…just plate it, and serve it with a smile!

If your child is missing her old treats: Give her G-free foods special names—the Minnie Mouse Muffin, or the Batman Brownie, or the Captain Hook Cupcake—so she will brag about the privilege of eating them (while making her classmates jealous in the process!). If you sell the G-free diet to kids when they are young, they will have a much easier time sticking to it when they get older.

STEP 3: DON'T LIE—EARN THEIR TRUST
WITH THE *TRUTH*

Honesty is *always* the way to go: Trying to hide this kind of critical information from your children will create problems in the long run. Kids have high levels of emotional intelligence, and pulling the wool over their eyes is harder than you think. The last thing you want is for them to be embarrassed or confused by their diet.

"We were just totally honest with her," Kathy Burger said of her daughter. "When she got the blood work done, we told Katie, 'The doctor did all those things so we could find out what's been making your belly so sick and what's been making you have diarrhea.' We tried to explain everything to her right away, and she was already upset by the diarrhea, because she was at the age where you would start potty training, but I couldn't start potty training someone who's having diarrhea fifteen to twenty times a day. So we just said, 'This is going to help your belly be better and help you not feel sick. You'll be able to wear big girl underwear and do all that kind of stuff.' That was all she ever needed to hear."

Stage IV: Getting Involved at School

The start of every school year can be a delicate time for G-free kids—and their parents. The chaos of transitions can make dietary restrictions harder to enforce, and you might occasionally feel as if you are reinventing the wheel every time your child moves up a grade.

STEP 1: TALK TO TEACHERS

At the start of each and every school year, you need to walk your child's teacher through the minutiae of a gluten-free diet. Make sure that the teacher understands the seriousness of the diet, and the potential consequences of not following it.

Classes, especially in elementary school, often have special events involving donuts, birthday cakes, and other gluten-containing food. If the teacher tells you in advance about these special occasions, you can be sure that your child has a treat of his own. Make sure that teachers understand how cross-contamination works, and also emphasize that the teacher should make an effort to keep your

---

Get It in Writing

Whenever your child moves up a grade, you should write a letter describing the dietary restrictions of celiac children. Send it not just to your child's teacher, but to the school principal, the head of the cafeteria, and any other officials who will be regularly supervising your child. Here's an example of something you might send:

Dear Mrs. Anderson,

My daughter Lucy has been diagnosed with celiac disease, an autoimmune disorder triggered by eating gluten, which is found in wheat, barley, rye, and some oats. Lucy must stick to a 100% gluten-free diet for the rest of her life. If she comes into contact with any gluten-containing substances—or even substances that have been on the same plate as gluten—she will get very sick.

I am making an effort to educate the cafeteria staff about my child's restricted diet, but I am relying on your understanding as well. I would be extremely grateful if you could inform me in advance about any field trips, birthday parties, or other special occasions that might involve food. I would also like to know about any art projects undertaken by the class, since many art materials contain gluten as well.

If Lucy does have a reaction, please notify me immediately.

---

child's life as normal as possible, rather than reduce him to his disease. Also make an effort to build a relationship with your child's teacher, and with other school administration officials as well.

STEP 2: BECOME A (G-FREE) PACK RAT

Even before sending your G-free child off to school, you should get into the habit of keeping backup meals and snacks on hand.

Make extra muffins and cupcakes and store them in the freezer at home. If possible, stock your child's school freezer with extra brownies in case of a snack or party emergency. Experiment with different portable snacks that your child can take on field trips and to after-school activities. If a treat is a hit, make lots more! Kathy Burger recommends having an extra freezer if you have the room—you can make it an exclusively G-free zone.

STEP 3: HAVE A CLASS MEETING

Turning your child's school into a safe G-free zone will not happen overnight. For more reliable results, you should try a variety of strategies simultaneously. One effective tactic would be to get a conversation started at school. Have an informal gathering with your child's class, and include as many different people as possible—teachers, administrators, cafeteria staffers, and of course, your child's classmates and their parents.

The topic does not just have to be celiac disease—you can address *all* of the food allergies that have been on the rise in recent years. Think of a fun name for the event, and encourage the person leading the discussion to speak in terms appropriate for the age group: "Hey, you know how everybody's different, how everybody has a different color of hair and eyes? Well, our tummies are different, too. To celebrate our special differences, we are going to have food day! We are going to make a brownie without gluten *or* peanuts—does anyone here know what 'gluten' means?" "Now can everyone say 'G-free'?"

Have the kids with allergies armed and ready and excited to tell people about their allergy. This strategy is particularly effective with younger kids, who are still bursting with self-confidence and love nothing more than to talk about themselves and what makes them special—so take advantage of their openness.

By framing food allergies in a positive light, you are teaching kids to tolerate, respect, and accept their classmates' differences.

With any luck, you are also teaching them to love and protect one another. If children truly understand how serious a reaction to an allergenic substance can be, they will look out for their friends' safety. My daughter came home from school one day and said, "Mommy, know what's cool? A boy in my class is G-free like you!"

Believe me: Kids get it!

STEP 4: WORK TO CHANGE CAFETERIA STANDARDS

If you are exceptionally motivated, consider banding with other parents and lobbying your child's school to serve food that is safe for children with a wide range of allergies. In the future, more and more mainstream cafeterias will be providing alternatives and taking measures to prevent cross-contamination. With a strong effort, we can help make that day come sooner!

In the meantime, you can still ensure that your child is getting a safe meal at school. Under the Americans with Disabilities Act, schools are required by law to cater to students with celiac disease. At the beginning of the school year, discuss your child's menu options with the school's administration.

Stage V: There's Power in Numbers

We all yearn for a sense of belonging, and never so much as in childhood. Joining a support group for kids with celiac disease can help give your child (not to mention you!) a much-needed sense of community and belonging.

STEP 1: JOIN A SUPPORT GROUP

Raising Our Celiac Kids (ROCK) is a support group for children and their families and friends on a gluten-free diet. Just about every major city in the country has a ROCK branch, and even a lot of small towns have organizations devoted to kids with celiac disease. (If there is not an association in your area, you could always start one of your own!) In case you were wondering: These groups are not grim at all. While the kids are off having fun in a safe, G-free environment, their parents might be swapping tips on local restaurants and grocery stores, or discussing strategies that have worked (or failed) at local schools.

If, like many parents, your schedule is too crowded for this type of activity, you can always find this fellowship online. R.O.C.K.'s Internet support group has been incredibly helpful to Kathy Burger: "I've actually never been able to make it to a meeting, but their e-mails are almost better," she said, "because they're constantly sending out information. People in the group are constantly asking questions and contributing recipes and exchanging ideas. [R.O.C.K.] makes you feel so normal—a reminder that somebody else is going through the exact same thing I am! Talking to other families who are going through the same thing is really what we rely on most."

STEP 2: RESEARCH SUMMER CAMPS AND OTHER PROGRAMS

If your G-free child is really benefiting from peers' support and encouragement, you could also consider a G-free summer camp—you'd be surprised how many choices you have! There are camps all over the country: in Georgia, North Carolina, Rhode Island, California, Texas, Michigan, and more. You can find more information on this Web site: http://celiacdisease.about.com/od/raisingaglutenfreechild/tp/SummerCamps.htm.

Stage VI: Encourage Your Children to Advocate for Themselves

The final step in raising G-free children is letting them loose in the world, and knowing they will be safe. This is where educating your child will play a critical role. The more your child understands about celiac disease and the specific principles of the G-free diet, the easier the "real world" will be to navigate.

One of the most important sentences you can teach your children to say is, "No, thanks, I'm G-free!"

Giving them the power to say no to food that will hurt them may actually prepare them for saying no to other harmful offerings later on in life. It takes confidence to do it, so allow your child to feel secure about being G-free. That all depends on you. If you are worried, panicky, or around-the-clock uncertain about food choices and social situations, your kid's going to pick that up. Be calm, confident, and proud—so your kids will learn to be the same way!

13

Throw Me a Bagel!

LIVING *WITH* SOMEONE WHO IS G-FREE

First, the good news: If someone you love has recently been diagnosed with celiac disease or a serious gluten intolerance, there's absolutely no reason for you to give up your morning bagel or go without your favorite four-cheese pizza from here on out (unless you want to!). But I am not going to lie: You *will* have to make some sacrifices to protect the health of your G-free guy or gal (GFG). No getting around it—both of your lives are about to change forever.

Will the journey you are about to take be easy? Not always, particularly early on. Yet will making these adjustments reap significant rewards in the end? Absolutely!

And if your GFG's celiac diagnosis seems overwhelming, try to remember what life was like *before* the diagnosis. True, you may no longer share your favorite fettuccine Alfredo as you once did, but there is a most important bright side: You also don't have to share your home with a person who is constantly sick or in a bad mood. As your GFG gets the gluten out, you will witness a remarkable transformation. No more unexplained migraines or post-dinner-party blues. Spells of irritability or long bouts of depression will become things of the past.

People living in chronic pain not only struggle to maintain healthy bodies: maintaining healthy *relationships* becomes a challenge as well. When you constantly feel imprisoned by your own body, you might have a harder time looking outward and focusing on other people, even the ones you love most in the world. Seeing the person through the pain is not easy.

I always joke that I have no idea why Tim continued to date me in the years before my diagnosis. I could never decide which quality was more charming: my bloated stomach, my frequent gas, or my constant irritability…Quite the catch, I know!

You will be doing yourself a favor if you try to view the new gluten-free diet as an opportunity to heal—not just the health of your GFG, but the health of your relationship as well. If someone close to you has been forced to give up gluten—maybe it's your husband or wife; maybe it's your child or parent, or maybe it's just your college roommate who visits for a week every August—make an effort to look at the diagnosis not as a curse, but as a blessing, because there are tangible ways to make your GFG feel better!

By cultivating a few qualities essential to the success of any relationship, you can serve as an indispensable ally on your GFG's road back to health. And who knows—you just might find that living with someone G-free actually is good for you, too.

Quality 1. Compassion: Don't Downplay or Dismiss a Serious Medical Problem

I've heard many people with celiac disease complain about their relatives' occasionally dismissive reactions to their condition. "Oh, it's just an allergy! You are lucky that all you have to do is give up—what did you say it was again? Glucose?" But let me tell you: While it's true that people with celiac disease have the unique ability to take charge of their health, giving up gluten is *not* a walk in the park. The sudden need to remake your diet—and your entire way of living in the world—can come as an incredibly traumatic shock at any age. What it requires of you, more than ever before, is sensitivity and compassion when the subject arises. Recognize that your GFG is coping with a fairly extreme lifestyle adjustment, and that your support and encouragement will go a long way.

Quality 2. Adaptability: You Don't Always Get to Choose What's for Dinner

From now on, most food choices in your household—what to eat and where to eat it—will fall to the person with the more specific diet. It is not uncommon to resent your GFG from time to time. After all, you may make a mean apple pie and your favorite taste tester is now out of commission. It may be helpful to spend some time figuring out recipes and restaurants that you both agree on. There will be times (many of them) when the new rules and restrictions will frustrate you, even if you are the most generous, easygoing person in the world. There will be nights when you really, *really* want to go out for pizza but know that suggestion won't go over well at home. If your GFG has celiac disease, reminding yourself that the gluten-free diet is not a choice but a medical requirement often helps. If your GFG is making the change for lifestyle and overall health, you might benefit from trying out the new diet yourself!

And if nothing else, there's always the next meal. Honestly, how many couples do *you* know who eat three meals a day together? If you work outside the home, you could try to get your gluten fix during business hours, at the sandwich place across the street from your office. I am not saying you will be denied gluten at dinner; you just might have ravioli less often than before. And you might have to give up your favorite flavored coffee, or invest in your own separate coffeemaker. If you are adaptable, you can make these minor adjustments without much difficulty.

Quality 3. Candor: Be a Gluten Guard

People with celiac disease must ultimately learn how to speak up for themselves and tell others—friends, waiters, in-laws—what they can and can't eat. But that does not mean you can't also speak up on their behalf every once in a while. Speaking from my own experience, I know that I am *much* more assertive on some days than others. Sometimes, I will go into a restaurant on a mission, giving the waiter a long lecture on the life-or-death importance of keeping any gluten-contaminated items off my plate.

On other days, exhaustion sets in, and I won't feel like launching into yet another superdetailed explanation of my diet. I simply want to sit back in my chair like a normal person and order like everyone else for a change. On those nights, Tim has become a pro at advocating for me (especially when I am pregnant). If I am ever vague or shy with a waiter, he will clarify my needs: "Just so we're on the same page," he will say, "she cannot have any marinades. Her food needs to be prepared in a separate pan that hasn't come into contact with any gluten. She cannot have anything but that chicken on her plate and the vegetables on a separate side plate. Thanks for doing that for her." He will basically fill in the blanks of all the advisories I *should* be giving every time I sit down at a restaurant. Two advocates are better than one!

If you are in Tim's position and find this role occasionally maddening, remember all that *you* have to gain from keeping your GFG on the straight and narrow. If your GFG's chicken is served with a little gluten in the marinade, you will *both* suffer for the accident. If your GFG is in pain for the next four days—too lethargic and cranky to get anything done—who is left to pick up the pieces? That's right: you and you alone.

And one more thing: Even as Tim serves as my wingman and occasional spokesman, he has also been wonderful at pushing me to become a more aggressive advocate for myself. Whenever I am inconsistent about describing my diet, he will remind me of all I stand to lose by *not* speaking up for myself. For anyone juggling the responsibilities of a full-time job with parenthood, these reminders can be *very* useful.

Quality 4. Preparedness: Never Leave Your House without Proper Supplies

People with celiac disease need to take a few extra steps before leaving home for any length of time—and in the future, so might you. You are a team; don't forget that. Remind your GFG to pack snacks ahead of time, especially if you are off to a long wedding, banquet-style event, or plane trip. Be on the lookout for your GFG's moods, good and bad, and fluctuating energy levels. No matter how many snacks you bring along, it can still be hard to sit through a long meal without lifting your fork. And if you are at an event where a great deal of alcohol is being consumed, keep an eye on your GFG. Alcohol lowers our inhibitions, and blunts our antigluten defenses. If your GFG is drinking without eating enough, the temptation to eat gluten might loom large. Do yourselves both a favor by remaining on the lookout for these occasional lapses. You won't regret it.

Quality 5. Open-Mindedness: Be Willing to Try New Foods

Would the word "quinoa" ever have crossed Tim's lips if not for my celiac diagnosis? I highly doubt it. Even eating whole-wheat pasta was a big deal for him back in the day. But he's an athlete, and I think he's really benefited from trying all these foods that otherwise might never have entered our lives. Yes, 99 times out of 100, he will still take the slice of pepperoni pizza over the gluten-free pita, but he's still really enjoyed learning about new foods—and you might, too, if you keep an open mind. To the greatest extent possible, try to treat the elimination of gluten from your GFG's diet as a learning opportunity, not a punishment. Eating a wider variety of grains could be great for your health, too, so don't close the door on new foods (however exotic they might seem) before you've sampled them. In most families, this introduction to new foods is most effective if done slowly, one unfamiliar ingredient at a time.

Quality 6. Cleanliness: Wash Your Hands and Brush Your Teeth after Contact with Gluten

If someone in your life cannot tolerate gluten, you might need to get a little more obsessive-compulsive about personal hygiene. Eat as many cupcakes as you want, but be sure to wipe the crumbs off your mouth or brush your teeth before kissing your GFG. (Some people recommend flossing as well, but let's not *totally* kill the moment!) And if you are about to bathe your celiac child, make sure you haven't just slathered your hands in a lotion full of wheat protein. You should also avoid drinking from the same glass if one person is eating gluten and the other isn't. (Need I mention "backwash"?) Be a little more careful in the kitchen. For example, never double-dip the knife you just made your sandwich with back into the peanut butter jar of your G-free family member. All these seemingly trivial actions can make a world of difference.

Quality 7. Selflessness: Put Other People's Needs before Your Own

People with celiac disease have no choice but to give up gluten. And whether we like it or not, we depend on our friends and especially our family members to make adjustments for us. There are lots of little steps you can take to help your GFG along:

- If you eat gluten and a family member does not, try not to polish off all the G-free snacks in the house—even if you can't find anything better to eat at the time. To stick to the diet, your GFG relies on a strong selection of G-free food available at all times.
- When choosing between a restaurant that does not have a gluten-free menu and one that does, opt for the place that makes your GFG most comfortable, at least every once in a while.
- If you are the head chef of your household and feel like making pasta for dinner, you might have to make a second meal for the G-free guy or gal in your life as well. You also might have to become more detail-oriented in the kitchen: Pay attention to which spatula goes into which pan, and be careful not to spread the regular jelly on the G-free bread.

In many ways, I look to my husband as an example of the selflessness and generosity it takes to live with a person on a special diet. Tim has gone to bat for me in so many different ways over the years, from advocating for me at restaurants to monitoring my self-discipline at weddings. Just last summer, I came home from a day of swimming with Grace to find a delicious G-free pizza waiting on the kitchen table. All his unbelievable acts of kindness have made a tremendous difference in my life, and our relationship as well.

Action Checklist

- Try to sympathize with what your GFG is going through.
- Get in the habit of thinking ahead, just like your GFG.
- Be flexible and easygoing at mealtimes. Accept that, from now on, most food choices will probably fall to your GFG.
- Develop a neat-freak side, for your GFG's protection.
- Learn to speak up on your GFG's behalf.

Show Your Gratitude

If you're the one who is G-free, you should always let the people in your life know how much their accommodating attitudes mean to you. Over the years, people have gone to great lengths to make me feel at ease in their homes, and I hope they know how appreciative I remain. Several years ago, when Tim and I were living in California, we became close with another couple. Early on in our friendship, before we knew each other well, I just mentioned *once* that I couldn't eat gluten, so when we showed up at their house for dinner, I was shocked to find an entire G-free lasagna made just for me! I was so thankful that I sat there and wolfed down half of that lasagna all by myself. I was so stuffed that I could barely get out of my chair—but it was the most fun I'd had in months!

My family has also gone heroic distances to make me feel normal and accepted no matter what. Whenever I am home in Rhode Island, my mom is always experimenting with new G-free dishes for me, and she invariably makes me feel totally involved and included in every single meal. She even has a special set of utensils just for me, while my brother has searched for new G-free snacks I could try. Tim's mom is equally welcoming: Every time we visit, she unveils another amazing new G-free treat she's found for me. The pantry is always completely overflowing (and so is my heart!). Even our dads know to keep the chicken and steaks nonmarinaded, and on a separate area of the grill—without being asked. I don't stop eating until we're back on the plane to New York!

Another night, when out at a restaurant, at a dinner hosted by a new colleague, I was, as usual, feeling nervous about how to survive the evening without getting glutened. But the moment I sat down, the waiter came up to me and whispered that the chef knew about my allergy and had prepared everything separately for me. Just like that, I relaxed and let myself have a good time. A few extra precautions on my host's part made that evening one of the most enjoyable in recent memory for me.

These types of gestures really speak to your heart *and* stomach, so make sure that your friends and family know how grateful you are for the extra effort they make on your behalf. Going out can be stressful for people on a gluten-free diet, so when someone assures you that the food you are about to eat won't hurt you, you can *actually* let go and have fun. It is truly the greatest gift.

So if someone in your life has just gone G-free, look at this lifestyle change as an opportunity to grow closer, to depend on each other more. You will find yourself more and more willing to make tweaks, because you want your GFG to be healthy and strong, free from pain. Once you are familiar with the grave side effects of celiac disease, you will do everything within your power to protect his health and safeguard his future.

14

Gorgeously G-Free

(YES, IT'S STILL POSSIBLE TO GET YOUR LIP GLOSS!)

Did you know that your favorite shade of lip gloss might contain wheat germ oil, wheat-derived vitamin E oil, or another concentrated gluten derivative? Ditto for your favorite shampoo, hand lotion, and even mascara. Just as gluten pops up in the unlikeliest foods, it also sneaks into a wide range of personal care products. It's used to bind liquids, to prevent powders from clumping, and to keep colors from fading.

Right about now, you might be thinking: So what? Isn't gluten absorbed exclusively through the digestive tract, and *not* the skin? Why does it matter what kind of hand lotion I use?

Unfortunately, the products we put on the surface of our skin have a funny way of getting inside our bodies. If you are wearing a wheat-enriched lipstick, you could be ingesting a little bit of gluten every time you lick your lips. If your hairspray contains wheat protein, as many do, you might be inhaling gluten whenever you style your hair. (I used to feel sick for a day or two after getting my hair done at the salon before realizing this was the case.) If your contaminated oats-containing body gel splashes into your eyes or mouth in the shower, you could be admitting a little more gluten into your system. If your hand cream contains gluten, you might be compromising the benefits of your gluten-free diet every time you wipe your mouth, or touch food shortly after.

And on and on it goes—even the products our loved ones use can introduce gluten into our bodies. Think about it: If your daughter has slathered a vitamin E–enriched moisturizer on her face right before you kiss her good-bye in the morning, you could be ingesting gluten from *her* skin as well. Or if your child is G-free, and your lipstick or lotion contains gluten, when you hug or kiss her, you could be unknowingly, over time, contaminating her.

Because, as you can imagine, these constant, tiny exposures to gluten can really add up (especially if you suffer from dermatitis herpetiformis or any other skin sensitivities), you need to pay close attention to the personal care products you choose. But there's no cause to panic: Being G-free does *not* mean living without lip gloss. All you need to do is follow the same steps you would typically take before sampling a new food. Surely by now you are a world-class expert at label reading!

Calling companies directly is also typically a good idea, but do know that, unlike food manufacturers, personal care companies are *not* required to indicate if their product contains a common allergen. Still, even if getting answers requires a little more persistence than usual, your efforts will be rewarded when you learn for certain that your favorite lip gloss or toothpaste is G-free!

Translating Ingredients

Before bringing home any new product, check out the complete list of ingredients, either online or on the packaging. You will recognize many of the off-limits ingredients (*triticum*, hydrolyzed ingredients, oats, barley) from your perusal of food labels. If you see vitamin E on the list, you need to find out where it came from, since most (but not all) vitamin E extracts in beauty products are derived from wheat.

Be on the lookout for the following terms in particular—they could all indicate the presence of gluten in a product:

- Amino peptide complex
- Amp-isostearoyl hydrolyzed wheat protein
- *Avena sativa* (oat) flour
- *Avena sativa* (oat) flour kernel
- Barley derived
- Barley extract
- Disodium wheatgermamido PEG-2 sulfosuccinate
- *Hordeum vulgare* (barley) extract
- Hydrolyzed wheat gluten
- Hydrolyzed wheat protein
- Hydrolyzed wheat protein PG-propyl silanetriol
- Hydrolyzed wheat starch
- Hydroxpropyltrimonium hydrolyzed wheat protein
- Oat (*Avena sativa*) extract
- Oat beta glucan
- Oat derived
- Oat extract
- Oat flour
- Phytophingosine extract
- Rye derived
- Sodium lauroyl oat amino acids
- *Triticum vulgare* (wheat) flour lipids
- *Triticum vulgare* (wheat) germ extract
- *Triticum vulgare* (wheat) germ oil
- Tocopherol
- Tocopheryl acetate
- Vitamin E
- Wheat (*triticum vulgare*) bran extract

Write a Letter

If you've taken this list shopping with you and you are still unsure about a product's gluten content, try e-mailing the manufacturer for answers. In most cases, you will get a response within forty-eight hours. You can write a simple message, along the lines of "Could you send me an up-to-date list of your company's gluten-free products? Any details on the sources of your ingredients would also be appreciated." Or better yet, go into detail about *why* you want to know. Companies will certainly pay close attention to a note like the following:

> *I have celiac disease and cannot tolerate any products containing gluten or gluten derivatives. I'd appreciate it if you could send me an up-to-date list of your company's gluten-free products. I would be more than happy to share any information you can send with the celiac community, so that others in my position will know which of your products are safe to use.*

- Wheat amino acids
- Wheat bran extract
- Wheat derived
- Wheat germ extracts
- Wheat germ glycerides
- Wheat germ oil
- Wheat germamidopropyldimonium hydroxypropyl hydrolyzed wheat protein

It is also important to check manufacturers' Web sites frequently, just as you do with your favorite food products. Many companies are making progress and listing gluten-free products in their brand. You also need to be on the lookout for changes in product formulations—ingredients often change, while the labels remain exactly the same.

Be a Beauty Supply Detective: Take It to the Web!

In addition to calling up and writing companies for information, I am constantly going on web discussion sites like www .glutenfreeforum.com to get the latest updates on my favorite products. Delphi Forums (www.delphiforums.com) has some useful archives with specific ingredient lists and correspondences between companies and gluten-sensitive consumers. CeliacNet (http:// celiacnet.com/hygiene.html) also has a list of G-free personal care products. Whichever online resource you use as a backup, please be aware that product formulations are constantly changing, so settle for nothing less than accurate, up-to-the-minute information, preferably direct from the company.

Beauty on the Go: A Survival Guide

The brilliant Emmy Award–winning hair and makeup team on *The View* has been amazingly understanding about my allergy, and I completely rely on their creativity, open-mindedness, and generosity. They use only gluten-free products on me, and never share my brushes. They always warn me before using any wheat-containing hairspray, or simply use alternative products that they know are 100 percent safe. Whenever they come to me with new products, their first question is always, "Will you check out the ingredients, so I know whether to try it on you?" I love them for it!

While I know that having this kind of relationship with your stylist is rare, I also know that there's no reason for you to risk your health every time you get your hair or makeup done. The key here?

BYOP! (BRING YOUR OWN PRODUCTS)

Until your hairstylist knows all about your allergy, my advice is to bring your own beauty products from home, especially on your first several trips. Until your salon stocks products that you can safely use, you are better off sticking with items that you know will not cause irritation. When you first sit down, before even getting shampooed, explain your allergy in detail. Ask to see the labels of every shampoo, conditioner, gel, spray, and assorted goop that might be used on you.

In my experience, it is best to do your own research. You are the one most familiar with the ingredients, and you are the one who may feel their effects.

When getting your hair colored: Before getting your hair colored, you must go to the salon for a "color consultation," where your stylist will do a patch test on you forty-eight hours before your coloring appointment. Have your stylist apply a small patch of color on a strand of hair right behind your ear. Leave the dye on the strand for what would be the normal processing time of ten to forty-five minutes. If after forty-eight hours you have suffered no adverse reaction to the dye, you can proceed as planned with the coloring!

When getting your nails done: I take the same precautions at the nail salon. On the rare occasions that I get the chance to sneak out for what I call a "Mommy Mani-Pedi" (Translation: While the kids are napping, I race into the nail salon and ask for hands and feet to be done at the same time, one coat, with a quick-dry coat on top), I ask the women not to use *any* lotions on me, unless I am already familiar with the brands. I feel much more comfortable bringing my own lotion in, or just skipping that step altogether.

When having a massage: Ditto for your trips to your favorite masseuse. Massage therapists often use lotions on their clients—it's your job to make sure the lotion used on you contains no allergens. I would definitely bring in my own G-free lotion until I felt confident that my therapist understood what was at stake.

When staying in a hotel: I have already mentioned this, but it bears repeating: Whenever you travel, you should take your own food *and* beauty products with you. Never rely on hotel soaps, lotions, or shampoos—they can all be potentially glutenous. Play it safe and travel with your own arsenal of supplies!

If you are unable to find the full list of ingredients, err on the side of caution, and stick with the products you brought with you. If you go back to the same salon fairly regularly, you could ask to leave your bottles there, or you could tote them along each time.

G-Free Products You Might Consider

You will actually be pleasantly surprised by how many products you *can* use. The following suggestions are not meant to make up an exclusive list. They are just a few examples of the many gluten-free personal care products available at the time of this writing. If you don't see your favorite sunscreen or shampoo on the list, don't despair: It might still be perfectly safe. If you are initially making the switch to G-free living, keep a notepad by the bathroom sink, or in your makeup kit, and jot down the names of products that you use on a daily basis. Take that list over to the computer, and get down to investigating!

GENERAL

Dove: Most Dove (www.dove.us) products—from deodorants to shower gels—are G-free. Dove has a policy of disclosing comprehensive information on any allergens in their products.

Herbology Beauty: Herbology Beauty (www.herbologybeauty .com) has a whole line of gluten-free lotions and creams that I absolutely love.

Keys Soap: Keys Soap (www.keys-soap.com) makes wonderful gluten-free and nontoxic sunscreens, soaps, facial washes, and moisturizers.

Gluten-Free Savonnerie: Gluten-Free Savonnerie (www.gfsoap .com) specializes in hypoallergenic gluten- and casein-free soaps and shampoos. The products are also free of fragrances, dyes, corn, and soy.

Pangea Organics: Everything in the Pangea Organics (www .pangeaorganics.com) line is gluten-free except the oatmeal soap.

Burt's Bees: The Burt's Bees Web site (www.burtsbees.com) has detailed information on this ecofriendly company's natural, gluten-free formulations, including a line of tinted lip shimmers. Some Burt's Bees products do contain gluten, so check before buying.

Dr. Bronner's: All Dr. Bronner's (www.drbronner.com) soaps are gluten-free. The vitamin E in Dr. Bronner's products is derived from soybean oil.

Neutrogena: If you contact Neutrogena (www.neutrogena.com), customer service representatives will send you a complete list of the company's gluten-free products.

Kiss My Face: Kiss My Face (www.kissmyface.com), which you can find at most health food stores, has a wide range of gluten-free products.

Whole Foods 365 Everyday Value: Whole Foods brand glycerin soaps are gluten-free, and many store employees can help you make educated decisions about other safe products as well.

Tom's of Maine: All Tom's (www.tomsofmaine.com) products are G-free except Natural Moisturizing Hand Soap Liquids and Moisturizing Body Wash, which both contain wheat protein. There is also a gluten fact sheet on their Web site (www.tomsofmaine.com/toms/ifs/gluten.asp).

HAIR CARE

Shampoo and conditioner: Most Dove, Garnier Fructis (www.garnierusa.com), and Suave (www.suave.com) shampoos and conditioners are G-free. All Giovanni Organic (www.giovannicosmetics.com) shampoos and conditioners (even the Golden Wheat line!) are gluten-free. Burt's Bees Grapefruit and Sugar Beet shampoos and conditioners are also gluten-free.

Styling products: Garnier Fructis and Pantene (www.pantene.com/en_US) hairsprays are safe and G-free, as are Dove Shape and Definition Mousse.

MAKEUP

Department store brands: Smashbox (www.smashbox.com; everything is gluten-free), NARS (www.narscosmetics.com; everything is gluten-free), T. LeClerc makeup (www.t-leclerc.co.uk; everything is gluten-free), and M.A.C. (www.maccosmetics.com; ask for a list) are all good choices.

Drugstore brands: Brands worth trying include Lavera (www.lavera.com; everything is gluten-free), Lumene (www.lumene.com;

Sharing Makeup

Just as you have to keep a constant eye on your special spatula in the kitchen, you must be vigilant about sharing makeup and makeup brushes. Some tips:

- Always have your own set of brushes. If you have recently gone G-free, give your old brushes a thorough wash. You might also consider getting a brand-new set.
- If you have kids who, like my daughter, love trying on my lip gloss, you might need to buy two versions of the same product. If Grace has just finished a graham cracker and then asks to put some lip gloss on, what is mine *now* becomes hers. I then label it, and keep the double beside mine so that next time we can get "fancy" together, as she calls it!

---

everything except Lumene Hydra Drops skin care products and Hydra Drops foundation is G-free), Neutrogena (ask for a list; most lipsticks are G-free), Cover Girl (www.covergirl.com; contact company; many lipsticks, foundations, and mascaras are safe).

Mineral makeup and natural lines: Mineral makeup—Everyday Minerals (www.everydayminerals.com), Bare Escentuals (www.bareescentuals.com), Monave Mineral Makeup (www.monave.com), among many other brands—is almost always gluten-free. Its gentle, nonchemical formulations are recommended for sensitive skin in general. Ecco Bella lipsticks (www.eccobella.com) are usually G-free. All Trucco cosmetics (www.trucco.com) are free of gluten and gluten derivatives.

KIDS' PRODUCTS

While wheat germ is a less common ingredient in products made for children, kids *are* more likely to swallow shampoos, soaps, and bubble baths. If your child has celiac disease, you need to take extra precautions against exposure.

General: The entire range of California Baby (www.californiababy .com) products is both all natural *and* 100 percent gluten-free. California Baby has a wonderful line including bubble bath, sunscreen, lotion, soap, and diaper rash cream. Always a good bet. Burt's Bees also has many gluten-free products in its Baby Bee line. Check the Web site for details.

Shampoo: Suave Kids Shampoo (www. Suave.com) is gluten-free. The Gluten-Free Savonnerie also has a number of shampoos that are great for kids.

MISCELLANY

Toothpaste and mouthwash: This is another area where you have to be careful, since we often inadvertently swallow dental hygiene products. Luckily, most big-name toothpaste brands—including Aquafresh, Crest, and Colgate—are gluten-free. Tom's of Maine toothpastes and mouthwashes (including the kids' flavors, like Silly Strawberry) are as well.

Sunscreen: Coppertone and Badger sunscreens are gluten-free.

Shaving cream: Tom's of Maine Natural Shaving Cream, Gluten-Free Savonnerie, and Colgate White Non-Mentholated Shaving Cream are all gluten-free shaving options.

Deodorant: Most Dove and Lady Speed Stick/Mennen Speed Stick deodorants and antiperspirants are gluten-free. Tom's of Maine calendula deodorant (in both roll-on and stick form) is G-free.

Lip balms: Burt's Bees; Badger Balm; Blistex (most varieties; check); most Neutrogena lip products; classic Vaseline; and most (but not all) types of ChapStick. Kiehl's lip gloss is gluten-free, but its lip balm contains gluten—see how careful you have to be?

Again, the above list is far from exhaustive. Think of it as a snapshot of all the beautiful possibilities out there—a springboard for your own investigations. I promise that before you know it, you will be gorgeously G-free!

Action Checklist
- Read labels of beauty products as carefully as you would food labels. Familiarize yourself with all ingredient names that could signify gluten.
- Talk to your hairstylist, manicurist, and anyone else who beautifies you about your allergy.
- Thoroughly research all products before taking them for a spin.

PART III

MORE GREAT REASONS TO GIVE UP GLUTEN

15

G-Free and Slim as Can Be!

After nearly a decade of living G-free, I can honestly say that even if I did not have celiac disease, I would still choose to be G-free. Why? This diet, which I originally went on for medical reasons, has benefited my body *and* mind in more ways than I could ever have imagined. Gone are the days of living off foods with mile-long lists of ingredients, or one-dimensional starches that left me forever craving more...without providing my body with the nutrients that it needed to thrive. I have more energy than before. I have more stamina to train and work out more efficiently. By default, when those factors are in synch, I tend to want to eat in a healthier way.

You, too, may find that by building your diet around basic foods close to their natural state—foods direct from the earth such as fish and meats, fruits and vegetables and nuts—you will nourish your body, instead of merely cluttering it with empty calories and unpronounce-able chemicals. Though it may seem like a removal diet, the G-free lifestyle will in fact open your eyes to the variety of nutrient-dense foods you have been missing out on. "If you look at foods in nature," says nutritionist Ashley Koff, RD, "giving up gluten is actually almost a nonissue. There are maybe five things you can't have."

We are always investigating the amount of memory our computer hard drive has, or how many gigs of music our iPod can hold, or how many operations our phones can perform, and at what speed—why not think about the foods that we put into our bodies with the same level of specificity? If only we demanded the same efficiency from our foods as we do from our electronic devices!

As it is, we obsess over fat and calories but pay very little attention to actual ingredients in the foods we eat, and the essential nutrients that they should be delivering. Somehow, we lose sight of the fact that, quite simply, some foods are healthier and more nutritionally dense than others. Some foods fill us up and leave us happy and satisfied; other foods leave us constantly hungry for more. Foods that carry maximum nutritional impact are crucial, whether you have embarked on a particular diet out of necessity, or by choice.

Most people can relate to episodes of overeating. Many times, you might feel a persistent dissatisfaction, even after a monster meal. Sound familiar? No matter what *quantity* of food you are eating, if your body is not getting the nutrients that it needs, it will continue to want more. Your body has an internal checklist of vitamins, minerals, and nutrients that it needs every day to flourish. If your diet is not checking off every item on that list, your body sends signals to "keep on searching," to fill those nutritional deficiencies…thus throwing us into "overdrive eating."

Once G-free, you are no longer simply robot-eating bag after bag of pretzels. You are examining every food choice, and measuring how those choices make your body feel. Soon you become aware of alternatives—you will probably even want to research ingredients in *more* detail.

Refuse to believe the myth that a G-free diet is a restricted diet. In reality, the exact opposite is true. Some people will say, "Oh, I am so sorry that you cannot have so many things!" or "Why would you ever give up everything you used to eat?" Don't be fooled into

G-Free Testimony

Rose Miller's story: After I gave birth to my son, I was trying to lose the baby weight, but more importantly, I wanted more energy. I just felt too lethargic. I was getting up at six to go to the gym before my day, and it was killing me physically. I have been a "dieter" for most of my life and I think I have tried them all...but this time, I was just feeling unhealthy and needed to get back to more natural—not processed—foods.

Instituting a healthy lifestyle is important to me: I eat healthy, drink lots of water, work out, don't smoke, barely have a glass of wine. The working out in particular relieves stress and makes me feel 100 percent better. I find it even more important to institute this lifestyle in my children.

With that in mind, I did a lot of research about "detox" cleansing. During my research, I came across a gluten-free diet guide and found it interesting. I have a couple of friends who are allergic to gluten, but I have another friend who is not allergic and still lives without gluten. She told me she started a gluten-free diet not to lose weight, but to gain energy—and she has a similarly hectic life. So my husband and I decided to try the detox with a gluten-free diet.

I thought we were going to hate not having flour, oats, barley, bran, and so on, but we both loved it. Sure, we missed some foods here and there, but in general, the diet made us eat smarter and healthier—straight-up foods. We had lots of options that we wouldn't have eaten before.

We have found some great gluten-free replacements like the gluten-free pizza dough from Whole Foods. It is so good and is easier to use than flour-based pizza dough. The pancake mix is also delicious—my daughter loves it! The diet has made us both feel better—we don't feel as lousy after we eat.

thinking that going G-free means limiting your options. This diet is about getting more, not giving up. If you are conscientious and do your research, it will have the exact opposite effect—of *expanding* what you eat on a daily basis. Many people eat a nutritionally flat diet of wheat, wheat, and more wheat: cereal for breakfast, sandwich for lunch, pizza for dinner. Missing from this food schedule is variety—and nutritional balance. Before going G-free, I ate only one or two grains, and a fairly straightforward repetition of meals. Even if I could, I would never turn back to such a limited menu.

To give just one example: If not for my diagnosis, would I have ever even learned how to *say* the word "quinoa"? I highly doubt it. But as soon as I realized how powerful (not to mention yummy) this food was, I was absolutely astonished. Was it possible that a single food could give me such a megadose of nutrients? How could I not have known? Why was I not demanding as much from my food *before* I got sick? This once-mysterious food has since become an all-star staple in my cupboard.

The secret to long-term health and fitness is not counting calories and fat and leaping on the scale first thing every morning. (I have done all of the above.) Though these numbers may make you feel more in control, the critical information is what's behind those numbers. You can get triple the amount of fat from a bag of almonds than from a bag of M&M's, but the nutritional content isn't even in the same ballpark. In terms of heat and energy burned versus energy stored, 2,000 calories is 2,000 calories. That said, eating 2,000 calories of junk a day would leave you with a significant mineral and vitamin deficiency—and a significant lack of energy. Eventually, your body is going to cry uncle. Going G-free forces you to step *up* and start looking at the big picture.

Once you begin selecting your input based on the nutritional content of foods, you will start to witness the incredible effect eating this way has on your brain, your energy level, your whole outlook on life.

Learning to investigate what you eat, Ashley Koff, RD, confirms, can work wonders both on your body and your overall well-being. "If somebody comes to me and asks about giving up gluten, I will say, 'Absolutely,'" she told me. "We are overwheated. We eat too many premade products. There are so many naturally gluten-free foods that provide valuable nutrients and offer taste variety. So avoiding gluten, and incorporating these options, can be a health-improving, absolutely beneficial decision," she said.

Even if you do *not* have celiac disease, the G-free diet is a terrific way to amp up your health regime by demanding more from your foods. You don't have to give up gluten altogether if you're primarily making this move to slim down. You can start by G-freeing one aspect of your diet—your breakfast cereal, say, or your lunchtime sandwich—and see how you feel after a week. If that inspires you to remove gluten from yet another part of your diet, by all means go for it! But it is important to note that going G-free will not, in and of itself, make you skinny. That is not what this diet is about. This diet is about making choices that maximize your health and give you the most bang for your nutritional buck.

Even G-free foods are not exempt from the nutritional magnifying glass. Is it better to have a pasta without gluten? Yes. Are there some that are more beneficial to your system than others? Most definitely. Simply grabbing a G-free pasta or bread without examining exactly what it will offer you is better than simply grabbing the old standby, but your investigations should not end there. Read the label, and consider every ingredient. People with celiac disease are already in the habit of taking these steps before eating any food, and I believe that this extra attentiveness does more than just keep us safe from gluten: It also heightens our awareness of nutrition in general, and makes us think more carefully about what exactly we are putting in our bodies.

"People with any sort of food allergy are unequivocally better eaters," said Pat Manocchia of La Palestra. "The consequence of eating the wrong food is dramatic and instant. With someone who is just eating ice cream every day," he went on, "they might not really know that it's clogging their arteries. But it is. They just don't have that immediate feedback mechanism as a guideline." Even if you are lucky enough not to get immediately ill after ingesting gluten, you might find that, after a G-free period of time, you feel more sluggish than usual after coming into contact with gluten.

The G-Free Lifestyle

I struggled with my weight a lot growing up as a child," Patrick told me. "When I went to college, I took dance and I started losing weight and got very health conscious. But I always still felt like I struggled in terms of digestion, and the food I ate never felt good—I was eating whole-wheat bread and things like that. At one point, I had a conversation with my sister, who is also very health conscious and allergic to a lot of things, and she suggested that I look at Dr. Peter D'Adamo's *Eat Right 4 Your Type* (www.4yourtype.com), which is basically a blood-type diet. So I read a lot about my blood type, which is O, and it talks a lot about gluten and that gluten causes a lot of weight gain. So even if you're eating relatively healthy foods like whole-wheat bread or pasta, the gluten could be causing you to gain weight.

"I decided to try the diet, and I found that when I started substituting gluten-free pasta or bread, I just felt better. I had more energy. I could focus more. I didn't feel as sleepy. I now get my eight hours a day and feel good. I feel more alert. I rarely get sick anymore. Before I would catch colds, and my immune system would go crazy, but now it's completely different. So, yes, psychologically, mentally, giving up gluten has helped. And physically, too, it's helped a lot. My weight is steady. I've been the same weight for the last two years. I haven't gone up or down. My skin has never been as good as it is now. I don't have breakouts anymore.

"In terms of digestion and going to the bathroom, I felt completely different. I felt so much more comfortable and healthy. I've been doing it for three years now, and every day I find something else I can substitute for gluten. People I've told about this diet, especially my family members, had no idea that gluten can cause weight gain or can affect people that way, whether you have celiac disease or not."

Patrick Cole, of New York City, who gave up gluten to improve his energy levels and regulate his weight, says that, after three years on the G-free diet, he feels immediate stomach cramping and intense fatigue after any accidental encounter with gluten.

Eating plenty of whole grains and seeds such as quinoa and rice bran—which are dense in nutrients and rank much lower on the glycemic index than your run-of-the-mill refined wheat product—is crucial. Low-glycemic-index carbohydrates, which release slowly into your bloodstream, provide a steady flow of energy over several hours, rather than the quick sugar high that a plain white baguette (which has a glycemic index higher than 100—and the index ranges from 14 to 103!) or chocolate chip cookie will give. Low GI carbs can also help prevent the storage of food as fat. In making the switch to G-free living, pay attention to a food's glycemic index. Choose grains that provide for lasting burn, and not a quick spike and then severe dip of energy. (See the charts on pages 193–96.)

Many of the general ground rules for carb intake apply to G-free carb intake as well: "Understanding how carbohydrates affect your body is critical to a successful gluten-free diet," says Ashley Koff, RD, who recommends eating small amounts every three hours to optimize metabolism and provide more reliable energy. "We absorb nutrients better that way," she said. "Breaking up meals—and especially our carbohydrate intake—puts less strain on our digestive system. Whether a food contains gluten or not, you really have to pay attention to the balance of carbohydrates in your body." By the same token, just because a food is gluten-free, you still should not devour the entire bag (been there, done that, will do that again), however tempted you might be. You are not exempt from the laws of portion control!

Like anyone else, you also need to monitor the nutritional profile of your diet. G-freers often have deficiencies in fiber, magnesium, and some B vitamins. Often, this is due to the fact that most wheat and gluten-containing products are fortified, and have vitamins and minerals added to them. Most G-free products, on the

Another Key Supplement: Probiotics

Ashley Koff also recommends taking probiotics, the good bacteria that are essential to everyone's digestive health. Merriam-Webster defines probiotics as "a preparation (as a dietary supplement) containing live bacteria (as lactobacilli) that is taken orally to restore beneficial bacteria to the body." It is, as the name suggests, the opposite of an antibiotic; it is a supplement that restores some of the good bacteria to our system that so many other foods are taking away.

"The right balance of good to bad bacteria—ideally about 80 to 20—is necessary for optimal digestion, absorption, and immune function," she said. "Antibiotics and other medications, as well as poor-quality diets, significantly reduce good bacteria in the digestive tract, increasing the risk of chronic flatulence, bloating, diarrhea, and irregularity. In my practice, I encourage an increase in food sources of probiotics for those with healthy digestive systems to maintain the good bacteria. For those with chronic digestive problems, I recommend a quality probiotic supplement to address their symptoms. For my patients, I've found probiotics to be the missing link in their nutrition plan which allows them to consume a greater variety of foods without symptom exacerbation."

other hand, are not fortified, since the fortification process can often introduce glutenous contaminants into a food. Therefore, Ashley Koff stresses the importance of making sure that you are getting the proper spectrum of nutrients on the G-free diet. "As in everything, try to balance your nutrient intake (carbs, protein, fat) and get them from a variety of foods," she says. Many regular G-full breads are fortified with nutrients, so when you exchange them for G-free breads and pastas—many of which are not fortified—you want to make sure your other dietary choices make up these potential nutrient deficits. It can be fun to do so; throw some pine nuts

The Skinny on Working Out

Often people ask me what I do to maintain a healthy shape and stay fit. Do I work out? Absolutely—it is my primary source of stress control! Additionally, my relationship with food has come a long way.

You are what you eat. Since hearing it in elementary school, I have never been able to get that saying out of my head, and I am thankful for it. It makes perfect sense that input equals output. If you choose grains and foods with impact and lasting energy benefits, you will be able to work out more efficiently over longer periods of time. "You are an integrated system, period," confirms Pat Manocchia. "You don't separate what you eat and how you feel from what you do. How you eat and how you exercise—these are not involuntary activities. Your diet directly influences the amount of activity you do and how long you do it."

Do I do push-ups? You bet! I also subscribe to the theory of the Push Away. When you are G-free, that triple-size burger and fries are off-limits because of the gluten content. That, on many levels, is a good thing. Not only am I getting more of what my body needs, but I am also avoiding foods that my system cannot identify. If your body does not recognize a food, it is more likely to throw it into storage, i.e., a fat cell. When your body *does* recognize a food, it will convert it to energy that you can use in your day-to-day life, whether at the gym or at work.

With a consistent level of energy, you might just find that you are more motivated, and more equipped, to "bring it" at your next workout. As Patrick said, "In the last two years since giving up gluten, my body has changed completely. It's almost like I want to work out *more*." I have had the exact same experience!

on your pasta or include olives and chopped vegetables in your pasta sauce. "If you are eating a variety of real foods," says Ashley, "you are probably not going to incur any nutrient deficiencies. But if you are living off packaged and processed foods—whether they are G-free or not—then you increase your risk for deficiencies."

As always, consult with your physician before trying any new diet. If you are already G-free, make sure that your doctor regularly runs blood work to monitor the level of nutrients in your blood. Keep an eye on those numbers and track them as you continue on your G-free journey.

If you have gone on the G-free diet with the ultimate goal of slimming down, you should also talk to your health care practitioner about an exercise regimen that is right for your body. When your blood sugar remains fairly constant—instead of rising and dipping dramatically as it would if you are living off pizza and pastries—you might experience a surge in energy and stamina. Use this energy to your advantage, because no healthy lifestyle is complete without a consistent workout regimen. Whatever you like to do—whether you are a runner, a gym rat, a hiker, a biker, or a swimmer—you might find that the G-free diet gives you more of what you need to cross that finish line.

As I have said before, the G-free diet is necessary for some people, and beneficial for most. When you go G-free, your awareness of your own body—and what exactly you are putting in it—increases. Those mystery 56-letter ingredients are no longer an issue: You will be focused on basic, satisfying foods that pack a ferocious nutritional punch. Your energy levels will rise with your nutrient intake, and your health will take the front-row seat it deserves.

Ashley Koff, RD, prepared the following chart for me. She drew most of the information from Dianne Onstad's *Whole Foods Companion* and George Mateljan's *The World's Healthiest Foods*.

HIERARCHY OF GRAINS

Type of Grain	What It Gives	Where It Goes	Health Ranking	Average Glycemic Index
White rice	White = refined; produced by stripping off the outer layer of bran; most nutrients are lost during this process (ex. magnesium loss 8× brown to white rice; fiber 5×)	Replaces wheat in couscous or cereal; risotto (arborio); rice cakes	Poor	90
White flour	Made completely of the starch of wheat (no bran or germ); high glycemic load carbohydrate; approx 80% less nutrients when whole wheat is refined to white flour	Baked goods, breads, flour	Poor	71
Semolina	Refined wheat flour (starchy part only)	Pasta, couscous, gnocchi, desserts, Italian-style breads	Poor	92
Couscous	Steamed, dried, cracked wheat; only contains the inner starchy part of the grain; similar nutrient-wise to refined ("white") pasta	Combined with stews; mixed with vegetables, nuts, and seeds	Poor	91

(*continued*)

HIERARCHY OF GRAINS (*continued*)

Type of Grain	What It Gives	Where It Goes	Health Ranking	Average Glycemic Index
Macaroni	A pasta shape from white flour or semolina (wheat) flour; *see* wheat and white flour for nutrition information	Typically used in pasta salads, macaroni and cheese, and casseroles; some gluten-free varieties available	Poor	45
Whole-wheat flour	Finely ground grains of hard wheat kernels (maintains the germ, endosperm, and bran); highly glutinous (hard versus soft wheat)	Baked goods, pasta, bread	Medium (highest level any flour can achieve)	71
Graham flour	Brown color; coarse; whole-wheat flour that has some of the nutrients (originally from the bran and germ) added back	Graham crackers; some breads—denser, darker wheat breads	Medium	Low to Medium
Rye flour	Sweet and tangy flavor; dark to light depends on how much of the bran is left (also dictates fiber amount); low gluten content	Dark, black breads (pumpernickel); crackers; pancakes	Medium	64
Chickpea flour	Aka garbanzo flour; good vegetarian protein	Small amounts as leavener in breads; thickens soups and stews; as a coating for foods to be fried	Medium	Low to Medium

Type of Grain	What It Gives	Where It Goes	Health Ranking	Average Glycemic Index
Cornmeal	Coarsely ground corn grain (best is stone-ground whole-grain corn; others may be nutrient poor); when cooked = polenta; well-balanced nutrient profile: minerals; B vitamins (but range of nutrients depends on type: enriched versus nonenriched)	Bread, tortillas, pancakes, tamales, biscuits, muffins	Medium	95
Bulgur wheat	Aka wheat pilaf; wheatberries that have undergone pearling, steaming, cracking—the cooking provides a nuttier taste versus cracked wheat	Tabouleh, salads, pilafs, soups	Excellent	68
Brown rice	Whole rice kernel (only hull removed); short, medium, long grain; only form of the grain that has vitamin E and maintains most of its B vitamins; excellent manganese; good selenium, magnesium	Desserts (pudding); stir-fries; pilafs; breakfast cereal; stuffing; granola	Excellent	55

(*continued*)

HIERARCHY OF GRAINS (*continued*)

Type of Grain	What It Gives	Where It Goes	Health Ranking	Average Glycemic Index
Quinoa	Not a true grain; soft, crunchy consistency; very good manganese; good magnesium, iron, copper, phosphorous; amino acids (complete protein)	Substitute for bulgur, couscous; hot or cold breakfast cereal; salads; cookies; pancakes; today quinoa flour makes gluten-free options (pasta, crusts, baked goods)	Excellent	51
Amaranth	Both a vegetable and a grain; strong, nutty, "wild" flavor; popped like corn, steamed, made into a flake, ground into flour; stays firm and chewy (versus mushy) when cooked hot; vegetarian protein source, notable for lysine (amino acid) content; contains fiber (more than wheat, corn, rice, soybeans); extremely rich in calcium, iron, and good protein	Pancakes, tortillas, grain medleys, cereal, salads; smaller amounts of flour used in combination with others when baking, owing to its strong flavor and for leavening purposes, but it adds moisture to baked goods; for nonrising products it can be a greater percentage of the recipe	Excellent	60
Millet	Toast in a little oil before cooking to release flavor; complete protein; good minerals (manganese, phosphorous); alkaline; fiber; silica	Couscous/tabouleh replacement; or cereal—cooked, puffed, flakes	Excellent	71

BATTLE OF THE NUTRIENTS

Nutrients	Quinoa (100g)	White Flour (100g)
Protein	13g	10g
Fiber	6g	3g
Iron	51% RDA	6% RDA
Magnesium	52%	5%
Potassium	30%	4%
Manganese	112%	34%
Calcium	6%	1%

Nutrients	Buckwheat (100g)	Semolina (100g)
Protein	13g	13g
Fiber	10g	4g
Iron	12% RDA	6% RDA
Magnesium	57%	11%
Potassium	19%	7%
Manganese	65%	30%
Calcium	1%	1%

(*continued*)

BATTLE OF THE NUTRIENTS (*continued*)

Nutrients	Amaranth (100g)	Couscous (100g)
Protein	14g	13g
Fiber	15g	5g
Iron	42% RDA	6% RDA
Magnesium	66%	11%
Potassium	15%	6%
Manganese	112%	39%
Calcium	15%	2%

16

The Autism Connection

We already know that consuming gluten can have perilous consequences for those of us with celiac disease and related autoimmune disorders. But could it interfere with the development of nonceliac populations as well?

In recent years, researchers have begun to examine a potential link between diet and autism spectrum disorders (ASDs), which have risen at precipitate rates over the last two decades. According to the Centers for Disease Control and Prevention, ASDs—the name given to a range of related neurological and developmental disorders, including Asperger syndrome and pervasive developmental disorder—might affect as many as 1 out of every 150 children born in this country today. How to account for these out-of-control numbers, and how best to treat children with ASDs? Experts are still scrambling for answers.

But there's one thing that we do know: Nutrition has a direct impact on a child's development. And a growing body of evidence suggests that eliminating gluten and casein (the protein found in

---

Casein Defined

Casein (the word is derived from "caseus," Latin for "cheese") is the main protein in milk, cheese, and other dairy products. Like gluten, casein is also added as a binding agent to some very unusual products, such as French fries, cake mixes, margarine, hydrolyzed vegetable protein, gum, chicken broth, vinegar-flavored potato chips—even nail polish and paints! You will have to hone your label-reading skills even more to identify this sneaky substance in foods and consumer goods.

---

dairy products) from the diet can have a beneficial effect on children diagnosed with ASDs.

The "autism diet," also known as the gluten-free, casein-free (GFCF) diet, calls for the removal of all the gluten-containing foods that you'd expect, but it also requires children to give up dairy products, including milk, yogurt, cheese, and ice cream.

But does it work? How exactly might gluten and casein affect children with autism?

While there is no direct overlap between celiac disease and ASDs, roughly 12 to 19 percent of autistic children have gastrointestinal issues, with frequent bloating, diarrhea, constipation, acid reflux, chronic yeast infections, and trouble going to the bathroom. A 2006 study published in the *Journal of Behavioral Pediatrics* interviewed 50 autistic children in New York and found that 70 percent of the children with ASDs had gastrointestinal symptoms, compared to 42 percent of children with other developmental disabilities and 28 percent of children with normal development.

Dr. Kenneth Bock, an internationally respected autism expert and author of *Healing the New Childhood Epidemics: Autism, ADHD, Asthma, and Allergies,* who sees between 1,500 and 2,000 children with ASDs in his practice at the Rhinebeck Health Center, has learned to pick out the patients with gastrointestinal symptoms early on in his treatment. "I take a very careful history," he told me. One clue is "when you get a child with a history of very, *very* prominent abdominal distension, malodorous gas, diarrhea, constipation, abdominal pain."

He went on: "There are also kids who engage in funny behaviors, like pushing their bellies against the side of couches or chairs, or lying on the floor in funny ways. They're probably doing this because they're in pain, but nobody's recognizing it. Those are the kind of signs that number one, make you think about pain, because the kids can't put it in words; two, make you think about information in the gut; and number three, make you ask, 'Okay, so what might be causing this?' "

Though there is still investigation into a direct link between celiac disease and autism spectrum disorders, people with both conditions are more likely than others to have damaged gastrointestinal tracts. In celiacs, as we know, the consumption of gluten prevents essential nutrients from being absorbed. Children with ASDs also have a profound reaction to gluten.

According to the "leaky gut syndrome" theory, some children with autism cannot properly digest gluten and casein proteins. Instead of passing through the digestive system as they would in a healthy person, the proteins in wheat, rye, barley, and dairy products break down into peptides that "leak" into the bloodstream of children with ASDs, triggering an opiate-like effect in the brain. (Numerous studies have found higher concentrations of these opiate-resembling peptides in the urine of autistic children with gastrointestinal issues.)

"You get these morphine-like peptides," says Dr. Bock, "which act kind of like opioids and make the kids almost stoned." The result can be a reduced attention span, impulse control problems, erratic behavior, poor language and social skills, and possibly even seizures.

While the evidence is mostly anecdotal at this stage, many parents of autistic children swear by the GFCF diet, reporting vast improvements—in their children's behavior, eye contact, and language skills—following its implementation. In fact, in a survey of over 25,000 parents with autistic children, about 63 percent of the parents interviewed said that the gluten-free, casein-free diet has resulted in either a mild, moderate, or marked improvement in their children.

"That figure is pretty high," said Dr. Bock. "You can't discount thousands and thousands of parents. You have to give them a little credence and recognize that there are some kids who clearly seem to respond to this diet."

Dr. Peter Green agrees: "There's no scientific documentation that the diet is beneficial," he said. "It's all anecdotal, but people swear by it."

The University of Rochester is conducting a double-blind controlled study of the GFCF diet in the treatment of ASDs. The comprehensive four-year study, which is sponsored by the National Institute of Mental Health, will monitor the behavior of preschool-age autistic children on a strictly controlled GFCF diet.

Until the results of this monumental study are in, many pediatricians still hesitate to recommend what they consider an unproven and unconventional approach, and many parents remain intimidated by what is by any measure an extremely restrictive, and often extremely expensive, diet.

Dr. Bock has a different point of view. "I judge everything in terms of a risk-benefit ratio," he told me. "For me, the hardship of a few months of a dietary intervention—and it does put stress on the family and the child—is entirely worth it when weighed against the chance of the benefits that I've seen in so many families." As proof of this conviction, he has started 4-A Healing Foundation (www.4ahealingfoundation.org) to raise money for families who might not be able to afford biomedical interventions like the GFCF diet.

"In this day and age," Dr. Bock said, "I think every child with an autism spectrum disorder deserves a trial of a gluten-free, casein-free diet. If the parents can do it—and hopefully they can with support—I really think it's worth it for most of the kids. No, it does not work for everyone. I wish I could say, 'Yes, your kid's going to respond,' to the parents, but I can't. Sometimes I have a greater sense than others that a kid's going to respond, but I always make sure that the hope I am giving is realistic."

Dr. Bock acknowledges that putting a child on this diet can be difficult and even heart-wrenching, especially in the first few days. Beyond the obvious reasons—the necessity of learning about an entirely new way of eating, the added financial stress of switching over to specialty foods—some children with ASDs can experience an almost violent reaction to this dietary change. That's because many of them crave precisely the foods that could be causing their brains to misfire: pizza, mac and cheese, and ice cream.

"When all the kids want to eat is pizza and grilled cheese, or French fries and chicken nuggets (which happen to be coated in gluten)," said Dr. Bock, "that's another big clue" that improperly digested gluten and casein might be having an opioid effect: The children are literally addicted to the foods that might be worsening their condition.

Many, but by no means all, of these kids can exhibit withdrawal symptoms when first put on the GFCF diet. "I always make sure I tell parents that they've got to be ready for the kids to withdraw," Dr. Bock said. "It's like they're withdrawing from a drug, and the kids can actually get worse for a while. They can get lethargic; they can get hyper, agitated—really, it's almost like watching an addict come off a drug. So if you don't warn parents about this possibility, it can be scary. But if you *do* warn them, if you tell them just to bear with it for the first few days, then sometimes it just breaks, and the kids come out of that fog. They lose the glassy eyes and that stare. They may look their parents in the eyes for the first time, or they might say 'Mommy' for the first time...I've heard stories that just make you cry. Some are dramatic, but some are just, 'Hey, it made my kid much calmer.' "

Dr. Bock also warns parents not to expect the GFCF diet to produce any abracadabra, overnight results. "For casein," he said, "you have to give it at least three weeks. For gluten, we say three months." But, he adds: "I usually see a change way before that. It varies, but it's not unusual to see changes in a week to a few weeks. But we do say three months because that is the outermost time."

For the diet to work, he emphasized, parents can allow no wiggle room. "I am a real moderate when it comes to integrative medicine," he said. "I try to make my recommendations work for my patients' lifestyles, so if you miss a supplement here or there, it's okay. But with this diet, you have to be extremely strict. If a kid has even a little gluten, it can throw the whole diet off; it can completely change the effects you are going to see."

Another caveat Dr. Bock was careful to mention is that doctors almost never recommend the GFCF diet in a vacuum. "I usually don't *just* put the kids on the diet for three months, or six months, and that's it. Parents aren't coming to me to do a scientific experiment; they're coming to help their kids get better. And most of my kids *do* get better, but I can't say that the diet alone is the reason. Because younger children tend to respond more quickly and fully, I often wait only a short time between various interventions."

Still, the bottom line is this: However inconvenient it might seem, however much resistance you might meet at your child's school, or even in the pediatrician's office, isn't the GFCF diet at least worth a trial? As Dr. Bock put it, "A parent of one of my patients once said to me, 'Don't tell me this *diet* is hard—autism is hard!' And I think that's an important point to make."

I couldn't agree more. If eliminating gluten and casein from your child's diet can even slightly reduce the severity of his ASD, why not talk to a physician who could help you make this change?

Resources

If you are interested in learning more about how the GFCF diet works, you can find all sorts of detailed information, both on the Internet and at your local bookstore. These recommendations represent just a small slice of all the information available to you out there:

WEB SITES

- Autism Research Institute (www.autism.com)
- Autism Speaks (www.autismspeaks.org)
- The Official GFCF Diet Support Group Web Site (www.gfcfdiet .com)
- Talk About Curing Autism (TACA), "GFCF Diet on a Budget" (http://gfcf-diet.talkaboutcuringautism.org)

BOOKS

- *The Kid-Friendly ADHD and Autism Cookbook: The Ultimate Guide to the Gluten-Free, Casein-Free Diet*, by Pamela Compart, MD, and Dana Laake.
- *Special Diets for Special Kids: Understanding and Implementing Special Diets to Aid in the Treatment of Autism and Related Developmental Disorders*, by Lisa Lewis, PhD.
- *Diet Intervention and Autism: Implementing the Gluten Free and Casein Free Diet for Autistic Children and Adults*, by Marilyn Le Breton.

Conclusion

One afternoon last summer, my family and I were sitting in the backyard of the house I grew up in. Someone asked my "Mama" how exactly she made her "meatballs and gravy." The question perked Mama right up. Though in recent years, she had become pretty weak and sick, this reminder of what mattered most to her in the world—taking care of her family—had an instant rejuvenating effect.

We all listened closely as Mama launched into step-by-step instructions. Had I heard her go over the recipe before? Of course. But this time was different. Every part of my mind, ears, eyes, was memorizing. Memorizing the measurements, memorizing the technique, memorizing *her*… as if, perhaps, it was the last time we would hear it just like this…

Mama smiled and energetically gestured as she spoke. She was obviously pleased with all the attention she was commanding. No doubt about it: We made one heck of a captive audience.

Then something surprised me. Right when she got to the part

about adding breadcrumbs to the meatballs, she turned, looked in my direction (as her vision had gotten incredibly bad), and said, "And Elisabeth, you can use something gluten-free so that you can enjoy it, too."

I half laughed and half cried as I took it in. Was it possible that even my Mama, the pasta master of Rhode Island, understood?

That conversation will forever remain in my heart and mind, as it showed me that even the most devoted, bread-loving Italian woman could get why I had made the switch. After more than a decade (and far too many holidays and Sunday lunches to list!) of feeling sad that I passed on, and could not enjoy, her lasagna or baked penne, my Mama understood that I was declining solely out of medical necessity.

I can only pray that the rest of the world soon catches up with my Mama! While we have made great strides in recognizing and diagnosing celiac disease, we have a great deal of work to do in the areas of labeling, price lowering, and safeguarding against cross-contamination. My hope is that future generations will be spared the torments that so many of us have endured on the search for an accurate diagnosis.

My primary goal, in writing this book, is to promote the awareness of celiac disease. There is a great deal that you can do on your own to spread the word about this all-too-common condition. The following are just a few suggestions:

Legislative Action

LABELING LAWS

The Food Allergen Labeling and Consumer Protection Act of 2004 was a huge leap forward for the celiac community. Under its provisions, if a food contains any of the top eight allergens (wheat, milk, eggs, fish, shellfish, tree nuts, peanuts, and soybeans), its label must reflect that. Unfortunately, "wheat-free" and "gluten-free" are not synonymous, and the new labeling law makes no provision for foods that contain barley and rye, ingredients just as toxic to people with celiac disease. The FDA is working on developing universal "gluten-free" labeling guidelines that are just as clear-cut as the "wheat-free" definition currently in place, but they have not devised the formula yet. The USDA, moreover, is not required to label gluten (or even wheat, for that matter) on agricultural products like meat and poultry.

One day, I hope people with celiac disease and other serious food allergies will be able to enter the grocery store without having to play Sherlock Holmes…A widespread demand for comprehensive gluten-free labeling could make the difference.

FEDERAL PROGRAMS

Since pharmaceutical companies have no stake in researching a disease that cannot be treated with drugs, we have to look elsewhere for funding. Increased private and/or federal funding for celiac disease research would be useful in fostering awareness.

Another idea: Many celiac disease organizations, on the local and national level, are lobbying Congress to designate May as National Celiac Disease Awareness Month. Write your representative in support of this important legislation, which is also known as H. Con. Res. 70.

Consumer Action

RESTAURANTS

With food allergies on the rise all around the country, more and more restaurants are beginning to cater to the diets of special populations. Stay loyal to the restaurants in your area that put *your* needs first. If more customers like you start speaking up, other restaurants will soon follow suit!

FOOD MANUFACTURERS

Lobby your local supermarkets and favorite food manufacturers for gluten-free options. If food providers see the growing demand for G-free foods, supply (and selection) will increase, and the prices will soon go down. Already, the demand is growing exponentially. In 2006, the market for G-free foods peaked at almost $700 million a year. Just a few years before that, in 2001, total sales were just $210 million. By 2010, the market is expected to hit $1.7 billion. These figures suggest that it is only a matter of time before even the most mainstream food companies consider gluten-free alternatives, and ways of preventing cross-contamination at every stage of the process.

Call your favorite companies and insist on gluten-free labeling protocols. Ask them to label all gluten-containing products, and even products manufactured in facilities that may have the potential for cross-contamination.

Education, Education, Education!

MEDICAL COMMUNITY

As Dr. Peter Green has noted, the rampant underdiagnosis of celiac disease in this country is first and foremost a "physician education phenomenon." Too many doctors and nurses are still not being provided with the research, and the myth that celiac disease is a "rare childhood disorder" still has far too much currency. Roughly 1 percent of the U.S. population has celiac disease, but *fewer than 5 percent* know it, and that includes those with the severest symptoms. We need to get the medical community talking about this increasingly widespread autoimmune disorder—there is absolutely no reason for so many people to suffer in search of a diagnosis!

If you can find no explanation for your health problems, demand the tests for gluten intolerance and celiac disease. Chances are your doctor will not offer these tests to you—you will have to ask. When the results come back, get a copy of all the numbers! Do not rely on anyone else to keep those records for you. Taking control of your health is entirely up to you.

THE EXTRA MILE

Talk to your friends, family members, and coworkers about celiac disease. If your child has celiac disease, hold a school meeting to educate teachers, staff, and fellow parents about the seriousness of the allergy, and the need to include G-free items on the cafeteria menu.

Do whatever you can to get the word out. Because so little research has been done, many people with celiac disease—even those who are suffering as acutely as I did—simply have no idea that gluten is damaging their bodies. If you have celiac disease, get your family members tested. Introduce the people in your life to great-tasting, G-free alternatives to their favorite foods, and let everyone know that living G-free is the way to be!

APPENDIX

RESOURCES

Books

GENERAL GUIDES

- *The Gluten-Free Bible,* by Jax Peters Lowell
- *Celiac Disease: A Hidden Epidemic,* by Peter Green, MD
- *Living Gluten-Free for Dummies,* by Danna Korn

COOKBOOKS

- *Recipes for IBS,* by Ashley Koff, RD
- *The Best-Ever Wheat- and Gluten-Free Baking Book,* by Mary Ann Wenniger with Mace Wenniger
- *Beyond Rice Cakes,* by Vanessa Maltin

Online Information

- National Foundation for Celiac Awareness (www.celiaccentral
  .org) is my go-to reference on the Internet.
- The Celiac Disease Foundation (www.celiac.org) is a national
  advocacy group that also has great information on the Web. To
  contact them, e-mail cdf@celiac.org.
- Gluten Intolerance Group (www.gluten.net, info@gluten.net)
- Celiac Sprue Association (www.csaceliacs.org, celiacs@csaceli
  acs.org)
- www.healthyvilli.com
- American Celiac Disease Alliance (www.americanceliac.org,
  info@americanceliac.org)
- University of Chicago Celiac Disease Program (www.celiacdis
  ease.net)
- North American Society for Pediatric Gastroenterology, Hepa-
  tology, and Nutrition (www.naspghan.org, www.cdhnf.org, nasp
  ghan@naspghan.org)
- American Dietetic Association (www.eatright.org, knowledge@
  eatright.org)
- Gluten Intolerance Group of North America (www.gluten.net,
  info@gluten.net)
- The National Institutes of Health (NIH) Celiac Disease Awareness Campaign (www.celiac.nih.gov, nddic@info.middk.nih.gov)
- Gluten-free "cards" for iPhone and iPod touch (www.appsafari
  .com/food/7201/gluten-free-diets.com)

FORUM

- www.glutenfreeforum.com

LISTSERV

- listserv@maelstrom.stjohns.edu

BLOGS

- www.glutenfreegirl.com
- www.celiacchicks.com

TRAVEL RESOURCES

- www.bobandruths.com
- Gluten-Free Passport (www.glutenfreepassport.com)
- Triumph Dining (www.triumphdining.com)

ONLINE GROCERIES AND FOOD DELIVERY

GENERAL

- www.glutenfreemall.com
- www.glutenfreemarket.com
- www.glutenfreemeals.com
- www.thefreshdiet.com

BY BRAND

- Amazing Grains (www.amazinggrains.com)
- Arrowhead Mills (www.arrowheadmills.com)
- Aunt Candice Foods (www.auntcandicefoods.com)
- Clan Thompson (www.clanthompson.com)
- Enjoy Life Foods (www.enjoylifefoods.com)
- Foods by George (www.foodsbygeorge.com)
- Glutino (www.glutino.com)
- Gluten-Free Pantry
- Kinnikinnick Foods (www.kinnikinnick.com)
- Namaste (www.namaste.com)

Grocery Stores

- Safeway (www.safeway.com)
- Shoppers (www.shoppersfood.com)

- Trader Joe's (www.traderjoes.com)
- Wegmans (www.wegmans.com)
- Wild Oats (www.wildoats.com)
- Whole Foods (www.wholefoodsmarket.com)

Products

BREADS

- Valpiform Breads (www.icaneatit.com)
- Ener-G Foods (www.ener-g.com)—preztels, pastas, breads, cookies
- Glutino (www.glutino.com)
- Food for Life brown rice or almond and rice bread (www.food forlife.com)
- Whole Foods Gluten-Free Bakehouse (www.wholefoodsmarket .com)

BREAD MIXES

- Bob's Red Mill (www.bobsredmill.com)
- Anna mixes (www.glutenevolution.com)
- Chebe Bread (www.chebe.com)
- Authentic Foods (www.authenticfoods.com)
- Whole Foods Gluten-Free Bakehouse (www.wholefoodsmarket .com)

CAKES

- Gluten-Free Pantry Chocolate Truffle Brownie Mix (www.ama zon.com)
- Cause You're Special Moist Lemon Cake Mix (www.glutenfree gourmet.com)
- Babycakes NYC (www.babycakesnyc.com)

- Authentic Food's Gluten-Free Chocolate Cake Mix (www
.authenticfoods.com)
- Pamela's Products Cake Mix (www.pamelasproducts.com)
- Whole Foods Gluten-Free Cake Mix
- Arrowhead Mills Cake Mix

CEREAL

- Some EnviroKidz (www.envirokidz.com)
- Bob's Red Mill Gluten-Free Oats (www.bobsredmill.com)
- Ancient Harvest Quinoa Flakes (www.quinoa.net)
- Bakery on Main Gluten-Free Granola
- Cream Hill Estates Lara's Rolled Oats (www.creamhillestates
.com)
- Enjoy Life Foods cereals
- Kay's Naturals Gluten-Free Cereal
- Nu World Foods Gluten-Free Hot Cereal
- Perky O's Gluten-Free Cereal (www.perkysnaturalfoods.com)
- Perky's Nutty Flax Cereal
- Ruth's Chia Goodness Gluten-Free Cereal

CHIPS AND SNACKS

- Kettle Chips (www.kettlefoods.com)
- Glutino pretzels (www.glutino.com)
- Ener-G pretzels (www.ener-g.com)
- Popcorn Indiana flavored popcorn and kettle corn (www.pop
cornindiana.com)
- Robert's American Gourmet Veggie Booty and cheddar cheese
Pirate's Booty (www.robscape.com)
- Lundberg rice chips (www.lundberg.elsstore.com)
- Barbara's Bakery (www.barbarasbakery.com)
- Blue Diamond Growers (www.bluediamond.com)

- Lay's Classic Potato Chips
- Pringles, fat-free only
- Tostitos Gold Tortilla Chips
- Xochitl Chips (www.salsaxochitl.com)

CONDIMENTS

- Amy's Organic Honey Mustard (www.rochebros.com)
- Premier Japan Hoisin Sauce, Teriyaki, and Ginger Tamari (www .allergygrocer.com)
- Bone Suckin' Sauce (www.bonesuckin.com)
- Hellmann's mayonnaise (www.hellmanns.com)
- Annie's brand salad dressings (www.consorzio.com)
- Mr. Spice Gluten-Free Sauces
- Natural Value Organic Gluten-Free Mustard

COOKIES

- Mi-Del (www.midelcookies.com)
- Pamela's Products cookies (www.pamelasproducts.com)
- Andean Dream (www.andeandream.com) quinoa cookies
- Arico Natural Foods Company (www.aricofoods.com) G-free, dairy-free cookies
- Gluten-Free Cookie Jar (www.glutenfreecookiejar.com)
- French Meadow Brownies and Cookies (www.frenchmeadow .com)
- Whole Foods Gluten-Free Bakehouse (www.wholefoodsmarket .com)

CRACKERS

- Mary's Gone Crackers (www.marysgonecrackers.com)
- Edward & Sons (www.edwardandsons.com)
- Sami's Bakery (www.samisbakery.com)—try the millet crackers!

GRANOLA AND PROTEIN BARS

- Biogenesis (www.bio-genesis.com)
- Lärabars (www.larabar.com)
- Bakery on Main Gluten-Free Granola Bars (www.glutenfreemall .com)
- Boomi Bar Gluten-Free Bar (www.boomibar.com)
- Enjoy Life Gluten-Free Bars
- Gorge Delights Gluten-Free Bars (www.gorgedelights.com)
- Mrs. May's Gluten-Free Bars
- PranaBar Gluten-Free Bars (www.pranabars.com)
- Raw Revolution Gluten-Free Bars
- PureFit gluten-free protein bars (www.purefit.com)
- Jay Robb bars and shakes (www.jayrobb.com)
- Elevate Me bars (www.prosnack.com)

ICE CREAM AND SORBET

- Red Mango Frozen Yogurt (www.redmangousa.com) is wonderful and completely G-free!
- Ben & Jerry's is mostly G-free, with the obvious exception of flavors like Chubby Hubby and Chocolate Chip Cookie Dough. Always check.
- Some Baskin-Robbins flavors are G-free, but order yourself some only if the tub is fresh and the scooper clean!
- Barkat Gluten-Free Ice Cream Cones
- Gaga's SherBetter (www.gogagas.com)
- Häagen-Dazs Sorbet (check with manufacturer)
- Edy's Grand Sorbet (check with manufacturer)
- Pinkberry (www.pinkberry.com)
- Skinny Cow, bars only (www.skinnycow.com)

MEATS AND COLD CUTS

- Jones Dairy Farm frozen sausage (www.jonesdairyfarm.com)
- Applegate Farms cold cuts and hot dogs (www.applegatefarms .com)
- Hormel "Natural Choice" cold cuts (www.hormelfoods.com)
- Most Boar's Head cold cuts (www.boarshead.com) are G-free, but remember—only buy them fresh-sliced if the person behind the counter has cleaned the slicer in front of you!

PASTA

- Tinkyada Brown Rice Pasta (www.tinkyada.com)
- Road's End Organic GF Mac & Chreese (www.chreese.com)
- De Boles (www.deboles.com)
- Thai Kitchen/Simply Asia (www.thaikitchen.com)
- Ancient Harvest Gluten-Free Quinoa Pastas
- Dr. Schar Gluten-Free Pasta
- Gilian's Foods Gluten-Free Pastas
- Glutano Gluten-Free Pastas
- Living Bean Gluten-Free Pasta
- Orgran Gluten-Free Pasta
- Pastariso Gluten-Free Pasta

SOUP BASES AND GRAVIES

- Emeril's All Natural stocks (www.emerilstore.com)
- Pacific Natural Foods Broth (www.pacificfoods.com)
- Maxwell's Kitchen Gluten-Free Gravy Mix (www.maxwells kitchen.com)

WAFFLES AND PANCAKES

- Van's All Natural (www.vansintl.com)
- Pamela's Products (www.pamelasproducts.com)

- 1-2-3 Gluten-Free Buckwheat Pancakes Mix
- Authentic Foods Pancake and Baking Mix
- Barkat Gluten-Free Pancake and Batter Mix

FROZEN MEALS

- Dr. Praeger's Sensible Foods (www.drpraegers.com)
- Amy's Kitchen soups, sauces, frozen pizzas
- Gorton's Frozen Grilled Fillets (Italian Herb, Lemon Pepper)
- Ian's Chicken Nuggets (www.iansnaturalfoods.com)
- Conte's Pasta
- Kettle Cuisine Frozen Soups
- Lean on Me Gluten-Free Quiche
- Martha's Home Style Entrees
- Mimi's Gourmet Gluten-Free Chili
- S'Better Farms (various)
- Starlite Cuisine Gluten-Free Taquitos

VITAMINS AND OVER-THE-COUNTER MEDICATIONS

FOR KIDS

- Bugs Bunny Chewables
- Sesame Street Complete
- Schiff Children's Chewable (www.schiffvitamins.com)
- Pioneer Nutritional Chewables for Children (www.pioneernutritional.com)

FOR ADULTS

- Pioneer Nutritional Gluten-Free Vitamin/Mineral Caps
- New Chapter Organics Vitamins
- Freeda Vitamins (www.freedavitamins.com)
- Advil
- Aleve
- Alka-Seltzer Gold

- GNC Mega Men and GNC Women's Ultra Mega (www.gnc.com)
- Rainbow Light (www.rainbowlight.com)
- Hammer Nutrition (www.hammernutrition.com)
- And many more!

PROBIOTICS

- Align (www.aligngi.com) Bifantis
- Jarrow Products (www.jarrow.com)
- Culturelle All-Natural Probiotic Supplement Lactobacillus GG (www.culturelle.com)

INDEX